Instructor's Guide for

Fundamentals of Mental Health Nursing, Edition 2

Kathy Neeb, RN, BA
Instructor, Practical Nursing Program
Minneapolis Technical College
Minneapolis, Minnesota

F.A. Davis Company • Philadelphia

F. A. Davis Company
1915 Arch Street
Philadelphia, PA 19103
www.fadavis.com

Printed in the United States of America

ISBN 0-8036-0729-6

Last digit indicates print number: 10 9 8 7 6 5 4 3

As new scientific information becomes available through basic and clinical research, recommended treatments and drug therapies undergo changes. The author(s) and publisher have done everything possible to make this book accurate, up to date, and in accord with accepted standards at the time of publication. The author(s), editors, and publisher are not responsible for errors or omissions or for consequences from application of the book, and make no warranty, expressed or implied, in regard to the contents of the book. Any practice described in this book should be applied by the reader in accordance with professional standards of care used in regard to the unique circumstances that may apply in each situation. The reader is advised always to check product information (package inserts) for changes and new information regarding dose and contraindications before administering any drug. Caution is especially urged when using new or infrequently ordered drugs.

TABLE OF CONTENTS*

*Please note that chapters 9, 15, and 22 have not been updated for the second edition.

LEARNING OBJECTIVES
1.   Identify the major contributors to the field of mental health nursing.
2.   Know the basic tenets/theories of the contributors to mental health nursing.
3.   Define three types of treatment facilities.
4.   Identify three breakthroughs that advanced the field of mental health nursing.
5.   Identify the major laws and provisions of each that influenced mental health nursing.

KEY TERMS
- American Nurses' Association (ANA)
- Asylum
- Deinstitutionalization
- Free-standing treatment centers
- Hospital
- National League for Nursing (NLN)
- Nurse Practice Act
- Psychotropic
- Nurse Practice Act
- Standards of Care

KEY CONCEPTS
1.   Mental health nursing has a long and rich history. It has evolved from the practice of very rudimentary skills prior to the time of Florence Nightingale, to the specialty area of nursing that we see today.
2.   Patients who have mental illnesses are treated in many different types of facilities. The type of facility depends on the patients' diagnosis and the availability of care in their community.
3.   The 1950s were important years for the field of mental health. During this time, the first psychotropic (psychoactive) medications were developed, which made it possible for people to return to their homes and communities (deinstitutionalization). These medications also allowed for more effective use of other forms of treatment.
4.   Nurses who are at all levels of preparation are integral parts of the mental health treatment team. Their observations, documentation, and interpersonal skills make them effective tools of patient care.
5.   A series of laws over the past 50 years has provided for money, education, research, and overall improvement in care of the people who are mentally ill. With the difficulties in the insurance and health-care industry in the 1990s, there is a tendency to cut money and services for care and treatment of the mentally ill.

CRITICAL THINKING EXERCISES
1.   The trailblazers were risk takers. One of the professional responsibilities of nurses is to try to give something back to the profession. How will you, as an individual, become a trailblazer? What direction should nursing, as a whole, take to strengthen the profession? What criteria are important when deciding what level of preparation nurses should be at to be considered specialists in the field of mental health?
2.   Laws have stated that people who have mental illnesses should be treated in least-restrictive alternative. Deinstitutionalization allows people who have mental illnesses to live in the community. For example, your city has just purchased the house next to yours

to develop it into a halfway house for women who have been child abusers. You are the parent of a 3-year-old. You are also a mental health nurse. What should you do? What are your *thoughts* and *feelings* regarding this situation?

3. Your employer has announced a change in the company's medical insurance policy. The company will provide you with a set amount of money for you to spend for insurance benefits. The three insurance plans you have to choose from offer an option for either family coverage *or* mental health services. You are a single parent who has two preschoolers. You also have a diagnosis of bipolar depression, for which you need medications, therapy, and periodic hospitalization. What insurance plan should you choose?

SAMPLE QUESTIONS

1. The main goal of deinstitutionalization was to:

   A. Let all mentally ill people care for themselves.

   B. Return as many people as possible back to a "normal" life.

   C. Keep all mentally ill people in locked wards.

   D. Close all community hospitals.

2. Another breakthrough of the 1950s that assisted in deinsitutionalization was:

   A. The Mental Retardation Facilities and Community Mental Health Centers Construction Act

   B. The Nurse Practice Act

   C. The development of psychotropic medications

   D. Electroshock therapy

3. The set of regulations that dictates the scope of nursing practice is called:

   A. NLN

   B. ANA

   C. Patient's Bill of Rights

   D. Nurse Practice Act

ANSWERS AND RATIONALES

1. Answer: B

   Rationale: The main goal of deinstitutionalization was to allow as many people as possible to return to the community and lead a normal life. Not all mentally ill people would be able to do that due to the severity of their illnesses. Not all mentally ill people needed to be kept in locked units then, or today. Community hospitals were to be kept open, but there were many state hospitals that closed due to the decline in census.

2.   Answer: C

Rationale: The development of psychotropic medications in the 1950s was a keystone in allowing people to return to their homes. The Mental Retardation Facilities and Community Mental Health Centers Construction Act came about 10 years later. The Nurse Practice Act dictates the scope of practice for nurses, and electroshock therapy, now called electroconvulsive therapy, was performed in hospitals.

3.   Answer: D

Rationale: The Nurse Practice Act, which is written specifically by each state, is the set of regulations that dictates the scope of nursing practice. The NLN and ANA are national nursing associations that set recommendations for practice, education, and the well-being of nurses. The Patient's Bill of Rights is a document that protects the patient. Nurses must know the parameters of this document for ethical practice, but it does not dictate the *scope* of nursing practice.

ACTIVITY
Both of these activities are fun to do in conjunction with National Nurses Week.
1.   Have students (and colleagues) research trailblazers in nursing and, on an assigned day, come to class in a costume or with a prop, and a brief explanation of the trailblazers and their contributions to nursing.
2.   Have colleagues dress in their respective nursing school uniform (or what remains), such as a cap, a cape, and so on; *or* have them bring in pictures of themselves from their "earlier years" (preferably in nursing school or at graduation). Post the pictures and have students match the instructor with the appropriate picture.

SUPPORTIVE MATERIALS
1.   The following videocassettes are available from the Alliance for the Mentally Ill/Minnesota, 970 Raymond Avenue #105, St. Paul, MN 55114:
    - "Asylum" (1989)
    - "With Open Arms" (1984)
2.   "Mental Illness: Awareness and Hope" (videocassette, 1988), American Mental Health Fund, 2735 Hartland Road #302, Falls Church, VA 22043.

REFERENCES
American Nurses' Association Certification Catalog. (1988). Kansas City, MO: The Association.

American Nurses' Association. (1988). *Standards of Psychiatric and Mental Health Nursing Practice*. Kansas City, MO: The Association.

Donahue, M.P. (1985). *Nursing, The Finest Art*. St. Louis: CV Mosby.

Keltner, N.L., Schwecke, L.H., and Bostrom, C.E. (1991). *Psychiatric Nursing: A Psychotherapeutic Management Approach*. St. Louis: Mosby-Year Book.

Park, C.C., and Shapiro, L.N. (1976). *You Are Not Alone*. Boston: Little, Brown, and Company.

Peplau, H. E. (1952). *Interpersonal Relations in Nursing*. New York: G.B. Putnam's Sons.

Shapiro, P.G. (1982). *Caring for the Mentally Ill*. New York: Franklin Watts.

LEARNING OBJECTIVES
1.   Identify three components needed to communicate.
2.   Differentiate between effective and ineffective communication.
3.   Identify six types of communication.
4.   Identify five challenges to communication.
5.   Identify common blocks to therapeutic communication.
6.   Identify common techniques of therapeutic communication.
7.   Identify five adaptive communication techniques.
8.   Define key terms.

KEY TERMS
- Aggressive
- Aphasia
- Assertive
- Block
- Communication
- Dysphasia
- Effective
- Hearing impairment
- Ineffective
- Language barrier
- Laryngectomy
- Message
- Nonverbal
- Receiver
- Sender
- Therapeutic
- Verbal
- Therapeutic
- Visual impairment

Table 2–1 helps identify the blocks and the effect they may have on the patient.

Table 2–1   BLOCKS TO THERAPEUTIC (HELPING) COMMUNICATION

TYPE	EXAMPLE	EFFECT ON PATIENT
FALSE REASSURANCE/SOCIAL CLICHÉS	"Don't worry. Everything will be just fine."	1. Tells patient his or her concerns are not valid 2. May jeopardize patient's trust in nurse
MINIMIZING/BELITTLING	"We all have felt that way sometimes."	1. Implies that the patient's feelings are not special

Lisa Anderson
Heather Arbury
Jim Borror
Maggie Spence

	EXAMPLE	EFFECT ON PATIENT
	"Why did you refuse your breakfast?"	1. Patient feels obligated to answer something that he or she may not wish or be able to answer 2. Probes in an abrasive way
	1. "You should eat more." 2. "If I were you, I'd take those pills, so I'd feel better." 3. "You ought to try a hobby."	1. Places a value on the patient's action 2. Gives patient the idea that the nurse's values are the right ones 3. Jeopardizes nurse's credibility if the suggestion does not work
AGREEING OR DISAGREEING	1. "You're wrong about that." 2. "I think you're right."	1. Places a value of "right" or "wrong" on the patient's action 2. Can seem argumentative 3. Patient may feel reluctant to change his or her mind because the nurse has expressed a value
CLOSED-ENDED QUESTIONS (*Note to teacher*: These are used in some instances in board review books. Alert the students that this would be a second choice if the observation was not offered before using the closed-ended question.)	1. "Can you tell me how you feel?" 2. "Do you smoke?" 3. Can I ask you a few questions?"	1. Allows a "yes" or "no" answer 2. Discourages further exploration of the topic 3. Discourages patient from giving information
PROVIDING THE ANSWER WITH THE QUESTION	1. "Are you feeling afraid?" 2. "Didn't the food taste good?" 3. "Do you miss your mom/dad?"	1. Combines a closed-ended question with a solution 2. Discourages patient from providing his or her own answers

STAGE OF DEVELOPMENT	APPROXIMATE AGES	TASKS/CHARACTER-ISTICS	EXAMPLES OF UNSUCCESSFUL TASK COMPLETION
PHALLIC	3–6 years	• Learn sexual identity and awareness of genital area as source of pleasure. Conflict ends as child represses this urge and identifies with same-sex parent. • Electra complex: "Penis envy": daughter wants father for herself; discovers boys are different from her. • Oedipus complex: son wants mother to himself; sees father as a rival.	Homosexuality, transsexuality, general sexual identity problems, and difficulty accepting authority
LATENCY	6–12 years	Quiet stage in sexual development; person learns to socialize.	Inability to conceptualize and lack of motivation in school or job.
GENITAL	12 years to adulthood	Sexual maturity and satisfactory relationships with opposite sex begins.	Frigidity, impotence, premature ejaculation, serial marriages, and unsatisfactory relationships

Erik Erikson (1902 to 1994)
Table 4–2   ERIKSON'S EIGHT STAGES OF DEVELOPMENT

STAGE	APPROXIMATE AGES	DEVELOPMENTAL TASKS	EXAMPLES	EXAMPLES OF UNSUCCESSFUL TASK COMPLETION
SENSORY	Birth–18 months	Trust vs. mistrust	Nurturing people build trust in newborns.	Suspiciousness; trouble with personal relationships
MUSCULAR	1–3 years	Autonomy vs. shame and doubt	"NO!"—Toddler learns environment can be manipulated.	Low self-esteem and dependency (on substances or people)
LOCOMOTOR	3–6 years	Initiative vs. guilt	Learns assertiveness and can manipulate environment (disapproval leads to guilt in the toddler).	Passive personality and strong feelings of guilt
LATENCY	6–12 years	Industry vs. inferiority	Creativity or shyness develops.	Unmotivated and unreliable
ADOLES-CENCE	12–20 years	Identity vs. role confusion	Integrates life experiences or becomes confused.	Rebellion, substance abuse, difficulty keeping personal relationships, may regress to child play behaviors
YOUNG ADULT	18–25 years	Intimacy vs. isolation	Main concern is developing intimate relationship with another.	Emotional immaturity; may deny need for personal relationships.
ADULTHOOD	21–45 years	Generativity vs. stagnation	Establishes family and guides next generation.	Inability to show concern for anyone but self.
MATURITY	45 years –death	Integrity vs. despair	Accepts that own life is fulfilling; if not, becomes fearful of death.	Has difficulty dealing with issues of aging and death; may have feelings of hopelessness

Jean Piaget (1896 to 1980)

Table 4–3 . DEVELOPMENTAL THEORY OF JEAN PIAGET

STAGE	APPROXIMATE AGE	EXPECTED ABILITY
SENSORIMOTOR	Birth–2 years	• Uses senses to learn about self • Schemata develop, which are ways of learning to assimilate and accommodate. They include the behaviors of looking, hearing, and sucking.
PREOPERATIONAL	2–7 or 8 years	2–4 years: • Thinks in mental images • Uses symbolic play • Develops own languages 4–7 or 8 years: • Egocentrism: only sees own point of view but *cannot* until age 7 or 8. This ability develops with age.
CONCRETE OPERATIONAL	8–12 years	• Ability for logical thought increases • Moral judgement begins to develop • Numbers and spatial ability become more logical
FORMAL OPERATIONS	12 through adulthood	• Develops adult logic • Able to reason things out • Able to form conclusions • Able to plan for future • Able to think in concepts or abstracts

Lawrence Kohlberg(1962 to)

Table 4–4 Kohlberg's Theory of Development of Moral Reasoning

LEVEL I: PRECONVENTIONAL			
STAGE	"RIGHT" BEHAVIORS	WHY WE SHOULD DO "RIGHT"	WHAT IF WE DO NOT DO "RIGHT"
1. Punishment and obedience orientation	*Do not do it* if it will result in punishment.	To avoid punishment	I will be punished and I do not like that.

2. Concerned with having own needs met	It is "right" if I (or if *we*) get something I want out of it.	To help me get my needs and wants fulfilled	I will lose recognition for the importance of "others."
LEVEL II: CONVENTIONAL			
3. "Good boy, good girl" orientation	"Good" means living up to what is expected of us.	Self and others think we are "good"	Avoiding "blame" is more ethical than getting a "reward."
4. "Law and order"	"Right" means obeying the laws and rules.	Maintains social structure	"Law" will have less importance than the will of "society."
LEVEL III: POSTCONVENTIONAL ("PRINCIPLED LEVEL")			
5. Social Contract	"Right" or "good" is behaving according to a general consensus.	We blend together for the greatest good and the welfare of all.	May become aware that "moral" and "legal" may not be the same.
6. Universal "good"	Universal rules of justice and equality for all prevail.	Live within the universal "good" according to own conscience	Few people reach this, according to Kohlberg; therefore, in this manual, the latest revisions do not measure this stage.

Ivan Pavlov (1849 to 1936) and B.F. Skinner (1904 to 1990)
Table 4–5   OPERANT CONDITIONING: B.F. SKINNER

SKINNER'S THEORY	EXPLANATION
1. RESPONSE	Any movement or observable behavior that is to be studied. The *response* is measured for frequency, duration, and intensity (e.g., chicken rings bell in cage).
2. STIMULUS	The event that immediately precedes or follows the operant behavior. The object is to find the stimulus that gets the chicken to ring the bell (e.g., food, noise, and boredom).
3. REINFORCER	3. A variable that causes the operant behavior to repeat predictably or increase in frequency. Sometimes this is called a "reward." The reinforcer has to be meaningful to the person whose behavior is being "operated" on (e.g., chicken pecks bell and food drops into tray. When chicken wants food, it knows that pecking the bell will produce food).

Abraham Maslow (1908 to 1970)
There are five steps to Maslow's Hierarchy of Needs. The steps are as follows:
1. Physical needs
2. Safety
3. Love and belonging
4. Esteem
5. Self-actualization

Carl Rogers (1902 to 1987)
Table 4–6   ROGERS' EIGHT STEPS

1.	EMPATHY:	"Walk in another's shoes"
2.	RESPECT:	Care for client as a *person*, not just a patient
3.	GENUINENESS:	Helper is a sincere/authentic role model
4.	CONCRETE:	Identify patient's feelings by careful listening and stereotyping.
5.	CONFRONT:	Discuss discrepancies in behavior
6.	SELF-DISCLOSURE:	Appropriate to situation
7.	IMMEDIACY OF RELATIONSHIPS:	Helper selectively shares own feelings
8.	SELF-EXPLORATION:	The more we explore ourselves, the greater/better the coping/adapting

(From Prochaska, J.O. (1984). *Systems of Psychotherapy*. Pacific Grove, CA: Brooks-Cole.)

Carl Jung (1875 to 1961)
Table 4–7   STAGES OF HUMAN DEVELOPMENT

LIFE STAGE	AGE RANGE (AGES VARY SOMEWHAT ACCORDING TO THEORIST)	EXPECTED PHYSICAL DEVELOPMENT	EXPECTED BEHAVIORAL DEVELOPMENT	POTENTIAL OUTCOME OF INEFFECTIVE DEVELOPMENT
PRENATAL	Conception through 10th **lunar month**	• Monthly • Cell differentiates(specializes) by the end of the first trimester • Intrauterine conditions of mother may affect prenatal development	• Fetus kicks and may respond to stimuli such as familiar voices, music, and so on	Threats to mother's health are of primary concern (smoking, drugs, malnutrition, and so on). Mother's prenatal habits seem to have a strong influence on the developing baby.
NEWBORN	1st month of life	• May have flattened nose, unevenly shaped head, and bruises from the passage through the birth canal; these physical characteristics will change over the first month of life	• Bonding (touching, talking, and so on)of parents and baby is said to be crucial to development of trust • Sucking reflex • Can see 7–10 in • Likes bright colors • Likes to be talked to • Prefers female voices • Likes touch, cuddling, rocking, and so on • Will not be "spoiled" by this attention	• Angry crying • Mistrust • Withdrawal • Stress, which slows further development

LIFE STAGE	AGE RANGE (AGES VARY SOMEWHAT ACCORDING TO THEORIST)	EXPECTED PHYSICAL DEVELOPMENT	EXPECTED BEHAVIORAL DEVELOPMENT	POTENTIAL OUTCOME OF INEFFECTIVE DEVELOPMENT
INFANT	2nd month of life–1 1/2 years	Infants are all very much alike (physically and developmentally) until the age of 10 months	2–4 months: • Begins to laugh • Follows people's movements with eyes 5–7 months: • Holds head erect • Turns head toward voices • Babbles/coos • Drinks from a cup 8–10 months: • Sits up alone • Says "mama" and "dada"; understands "no" and "bye-bye"	• Poor parent-child relationship can lead to mistrust and poor self-concept • Failure-to-thrive syndrome • Separation anxiety
TODDLER	1–3 years	• Long trunk • Short legs • Brain about 3/4 of full size in order to be able to support future growth and development • Walking	• Toilet training • Learning sex roles by copying behaviors of same-sex parent • Self-centered • Does not share • Wants things *now* • Both boys and girls are learning **autonomy** (independence)by using the word "no" • **Assimilation**, which is taking in and processing of information via the senses • **Accommodation**, which is the ability to adjust to new information or situations	• Anger • Regression • Revert to infant-age behaviors
PRESCHOOL (EARLY CHILDHOOD)	3–6 years	• Medical and dental examinations are important • Nutrition can be challenging—children are starting to pick and choose their favorite foods. This is the time to start teaching good nutrition. • Lead poisoning is still a threat. It tastes sweet and may still be found in some older plumbing or in old paint layers in housing units	• Cognitive development is a primary activity • Many questions; "why" is a frequently used word • Socializes • Play is important for self-expression and anxiety relief • Reading is the best parent-child activity • Aggressive behavior (roughhousing) • Active imagination can lead to nightmares • Mixed feelings about going to school	• Enuresis is the involuntary bedwetting in preschool and school-age children who have been toilet trained (often due to poor personal relationships) • Encopresis is involuntary bowel movements in the same situation as enuresis

LIFE STAGE	AGE RANGE (AGES VARY SOMEWHAT ACCORDING TO THEORIST)	EXPECTED PHYSICAL DEVELOPMENT	EXPECTED BEHAVIORAL DEVELOPMENT	POTENTIAL OUTCOME OF INEFFECTIVE DEVELOPMENT
SCHOOL AGE	6–12 years	<ul><li>Body thins out and growth slows temporarily</li><li>Lose baby teeth and gain permanent teeth</li><li>By age 6, brain is almost full size. The neurological system develops from the head down</li><li>By age 6 or 7, vision is at its peak</li><li>Vision and hearing screening is usually begun by the time the child enters school</li><li>Agility increases</li><li>Scoliosis (lateral curvature of the spine) screening may be encouraged</li><li>Late childhood (10–11-years-old) sees the beginning of sexual development, especially in girls. Females at this stage mature about 2 years ahead of males</li><li>Colds are frequent due to social habits</li></ul>	<ul><li>Learning to share</li><li>Forms friendships with same-sex friends</li><li>Peer group activities (secret clubs and so on)</li><li>Begins to show acceptance of moral issues by questions and discussions</li><li>Reversibility: the ability to put things in an order or sequence or to group things according to common traits</li></ul>	<ul><li>Shyness/fear of school if trust and autonomy have not developed fully. May be a result of not being included in peer groups; has been defined as a "silent prison."</li><li>Gangs can be the result of negative types of peer groups</li><li>Stuttering is repetitive or prolonged sounds or speech flow that is interrupted. Seems to occur four times more often in males. May be stress related.</li><li>Accidents are the leading cause of death in children. Teaching safety to families and children is important.</li><li>Child abuse/neglect are noted more frequently. *All health-care personnel have the duty to report abuse or suspected abuse.* Abuse will be discussed in more detail in Chapters 5 and 21.</li></ul>
ADOLESCENT	12–18 years	<ul><li>Growth spurt (musculoskeletal system)</li><li>Endocrine system maturing (hormones)</li><li>Secondary sex characteristics develop (facial and underarm hair, males' shoulders broaden, females' hips broaden and breasts develop, and so on)</li><li>**Puberty** means that the individual is capable of reproducing</li><li>**Menarche** is a female's first menstrual period, which happens around age 11–15. It is important to know that nutrition and exercise affect this.</li></ul>	<ul><li>Learns independence</li><li>Learns self-sufficiency</li><li>Learns new social roles</li><li>Mood swings</li><li>Boredom</li><li>Introspective</li><li>Preoccupied with body image</li><li>Own "language"</li><li>Peer group very important—teens need intimacy</li><li>Talking on phone for hours</li><li>Possible experimentation with alcohol, drugs, and sex</li><li>Communication between parent and adolescent is crucial</li></ul>	<ul><li>Anorexia and bulimia are frequent dangers for males, as well as females; usually are from white, middle-class families (Kalman and Waughfield, 1993)</li><li>Males who mature later seem to have the hardest time adjusting</li><li>Suicide is a major concern for this age group, usually because they feel unimportant and not taken seriously by adults</li></ul>

LIFE STAGE	AGE RANGE (AGES VARY SOMEWHAT ACCORDING TO THEORIST)	EXPECTED PHYSICAL DEVELOPMENT	EXPECTED BEHAVIORAL DEVELOPMENT	POTENTIAL OUTCOME OF INEFFECTIVE DEVELOPMENT
YOUNG ADULT	18–35 years	• Body usually in optimal physical condition	• Intimacy is the main task to accomplish • Schooling and career planning are important • Marriage and family decisions are made	• There are many choices in this stage that affect the life of a young adult. Ineffective completion of parts of the young adult and adult stages may affect how he or she ages and prepares for death. Not all theorists agree on these stages.
ADULT	30–60 years	• Gradual decline in hearing and visual acuity • Body beginning to shorten somewhat as musculature and bone structure change • Lung and cardiac capacity beginning to decrease somewhat	• Generativity, or passing down values and skills to the next generation (personally and professionally) is a major task of the adult	
OLDER ADULT	60 years through death	• Visual and hearing acuity continue to decline • Body becomes susceptible to an increasing number of physical and emotional illnesses	• Accept limits on independence and physical ability • Accept the idea of death and begin preparing for it • Accept retirement • Stress increases throughout the life span	• Fear of death and dying • Difficulty with retirement because identity is often associated with career • Depression relating to aging, loss of friends, and so on

Table 4–8   FIVE STAGES OF GRIEF/DEATH AND DYING BY DR. ELIZABETH KÜBLER-ROSS

STAGE	KEY WORDS	EXPECTED BEHAVIORS
DENIAL	"Not me!"	Refuses to believe that death is coming; states, "That doctor doesn't know what he or she is talking about!"
ANGER	"Why me?"	Expresses envy, resentment, and frustration with younger people/those who are not dying
BARGAINING	"If I could have one more chance…"	May become very religious or "good" in an effort to gain another chance at life or more time to live
GRIEF/DEPRESSION	Realizes that "bargaining" is not working and death is approaching	Becomes depressed and weepy; may "give up", quit taking medications, quit eating, and so forth

29

ACCEPTANCE	"OK...but I don't have to like it!"	Enters a state of expectation; may begin to call family members near; needs to complete "unfinished business"; prepares spiritually to die

KEY CONCEPTS

1. There are many theories about personality development in human beings. These are only theories, but there are strong indications of validity in them all. It is necessary for the licensed practical nurse/licensed vocational nurse (LPN/LVN) to have a working knowledge of some of the more commonly accepted theories of human development throughout the life span.

2. Dr. Elisabeth Kübler-Ross has developed a theory of five stages that people go through when they are grieving or dying. These stages also apply to their significant others. Although others have presented theories on this topic, hers remains the most commonly accepted theory in nursing.

3. Each person is unique and goes through stages of development or grief at his or her own pace. These theories are guidelines to help us understand what our patients may be experience as they go through certain stages in their lives.

CRITICAL THINKING EXERCISES

1. Your patient is in a monogamous homosexual relationship and is in the final stage of life. Death is imminent, but the patient is still alert and oriented. Family and partner are in the room. The patient asks you to ask the physician to "put me to sleep." The patient's partner weeps but supports the request; the family members threaten to sue if the physician does "any such thing." What are your thoughts about euthanasia? What are your feelings about euthanasia? What will you do to help the patient? The family? The partner? What if this was your parent or child who was about to die? What would you think and feel then?

SAMPLE QUESTIONS

1. Your little 4-year-old patient comes in to the clinic with her father. She is being checked for a recurring ear infection. As you prepare her to see the physician, she says, "I love my daddy. I'm going to marry him like Mommy someday!" Which one of Freud's stages of development is she most likely demonstrating?

   A. Genital

   B. Oral

   C. Anal

   D. Phallic

2. Patient Y is 20-years-old. Y is a perfectionist and very routine oriented. Freudian theorists would say that patient Y did not successfully complete which of the following stages of development?

   A. Genital

   B. Oral

C. Anal

D. Phallic

3. Patient Y (from question 2) is being treated by a behavioral psychologist. When patient Y begins to miss meals and activities due to the need to complete routines perfectly, staff members should intervene. Patient Y failed to come to dinner on your shift. You go to check and see Y carefully placing personal items in a special place in the bathroom. Your best response to Y from a behavioral and therapeutic background could be:

A. "Y, where were you at dinner tonight?"

B. "Y, you blew it. You didn't come to dinner and you know what that means—no pass for the weekend."

C. "Y, I am just here to remind you it is dinner time."

D. "Y, it is not appropriate to miss dinner. What is the consequence for that, according to your care plan?"

ANSWERS AND RATIONALES
1. Answer: D

Rationale: She is demonstrating the Electra complex, which is part of the phallic stage of Freud's developmental stages.

2. Answer: C

Rationale: Unsuccessful completion of the anal stage would lead to these behaviors and to more serious disorders, according to psychoanalytic theory. These people would be termed "anal retentive" in some social and professional circles today.

3. Answer: D

Rationale: This option states that Y's behavior is not appropriate and lets Y tell you that the consequences have been discussed. Y is able to make a choice. Options A and B sound harsh and threatening, and are not helpful forms of communicating. Option C is very close to letting the nurse "care-take" for Y. In behavior modification, Y would most likely be responsible for his or her own actions and choices.

ACTIVITY
1. If your school has a Child Development program or something similar, collaborate with the program to observe them as they work with their children. If this includes a buddy system off-site, try to arrange that as a clinical or classroom day for your class. Have the nursing students file a brief account of the similarities and differences they observe.

SUPPORTIVE MATERIALS
1. "Eight Stages of Human Life" (Filmstrip, 1980), Human Relations Media, 175 Tomkins Avenue, Pleasantville, NY 10570.

REFERENCES

Crawford, A.L., and Kilander, V.C. (1985). *Psychiatric and Mental Health Nursing*, 6th ed. Philadelphia: F.A. Davis Company.

Dennis, L.B., and Hassol, J. (1983). *Introduction to Human Development and Health Issues*. Philadelphia: W.B. Saunders.

Erikson, E.H. (1977). *Toys and Reasons*. New York: W.W. Norton and Company.

Kalman, N., and Waughfield, C.G. (1993). *Mental Health Concepts*, 3rd ed. Albany, NY: Delmar.

Milliken, M.E. (1993). *Understanding Human Behavior*, 5th ed. Albany, NY: Delmar.

Prochaska, J.O. (1984). *Systems of Psychotherapy*. Pacific Grove, CA: Brooks-Cole Publishing.

Rubin, Z., Peplau, L., and Salovey, P. (1993). *Psychology*. Boston: Houghton-Mifflin.

Shives, L.R. (1994). *Basic Concepts of Psychiatric-Mental Health Nursing*, 3rd ed. Philadelphia: J.B. Lippincott.

LEARNING OBJECTIVES
1.   Define culture.
2.   Define religion.
3.   Define ethnicity.
4.   Identify parenting styles.
5.   Differentiate between abuse and neglect.
6.   Define stereotype.
7.   Define prejudice.

KEY TERMS
- Abuse
- Culture
- Economic
- Ethnicity
- Ethnocentricism
- Prejudice
- Religion
- Stereotype

Culture
Culture is a term that gets misused. It is a shared way of life and the combination of traditions and beliefs that makes a group of people bond together (also see Chapter 3). Culture is *not* based on a person's skin color or country of origin.

Religious beliefs are often included in discussions of culture; however, it is important to note that the religion is *not* usually considered the culture.

Religion is a person's belief of some higher power. It involves a very strong belief system; so strong that people have fought wars over religion and it is often the subject of **stereotype**. A stereotype is a fixed notion or conviction (Merriam-Webster, 1994) about a group of people or a situation. Organized religions usually involve rituals or worship services.

Native-Americans worship different gods or spirits. For example, certain numbers are considered sacred and special qualities are attributed to the four directions of north, south, east, and west. Of course, all Native Americans cannot be classified into one large group; there are many Native-American nations and tribes, and each have their own sets of beliefs.

Spirituality and religion may be extremely important to some of your patients and unimportant to others.

Ethnicity
Ethnicity defines a person's more personal traits. Language, country of origin, and skin color are all part of one's ethnicity. There can be many different ethnic groups within a culture.

Education helps to eliminate **prejudice**, which is the prejudgment of a person or situation before all of the facts are known.

The hurt of prejudice has led to an emergence of **ethnocentrism**, which is people believing that their particular ethnic group has rights and benefits over and above the rights of others. Gangs, supremacist groups, and terrorist groups may have had their roots in hate and prejudice. People learn by sharing with others. It is much better to ask a person about something you do not know, than to make an assumption about it. That is a stereotype and can end a helping relationship (Galanti, 1991).

Economic

A study done by Eron and Peterson in 1982 found that the lower the socioeconomic status, the higher the incidence of abnormal behavior in U.S. society. Though, even this is not a statement that is accurate in all cases. This study showed that the conclusion applied more strongly to schizophrenia than it did to mood disorders. The implication is that there are always other variables besides socioeconomic factors. For example, people who live in poverty or underprivileged circumstances will very likely have greater stressors than others. So, is it socioeconomic status or stress that leads to the disorder?

Abuse

Abuse is misuse of a person, substance, or situation. Sometimes people say that they cannot be abusing, as they consider themselves to be knowledgeable of what they are doing. This is not true. Anyone who misuses or overuses a substance, a situation (such as gambling or power), or another person is being abusive.

Poor Parenting

Diana Baumrind (1971) has developed a classification of types of parents. They are described as follows:
1.   *Authoritarian parent*: This parent sets up very strict rules. The child has little or no voice in family decisions. This can lead to a rebellious and hostile child who enters adulthood as angry, violent, unwilling to obey laws, and unable to make consistent decisions.
2.   *Authoritative parent*: This parenting style has firm and consistent rules and limits. This style, however, allows for discussion and occasional flexibility of the rules, according to special circumstances. Children are allowed some freedom, within set limits, and some voice in decisions.
3.   *Permissive parent*: This parenting style provides little structure and few guidelines. The child is not sure of the boundaries. If children do not learn boundaries, it becomes difficult to learn how to control themselves and how to behave in certain situations. This parent may be in danger of being accused of neglect.

KEY CONCEPTS
1.   Culture, ethnicity, and religion are basic human experiences that are deeply rooted. They are not "good" or "bad"; they are different for each individual or group of individuals who claim membership in that culture, ethnic group, or religion.
2.   People are much more alike than they are different. It is important for nurses to concentrate on the similarities among people and to be comfortable asking questions about the background of patients and coworkers. Role-modeling cooperative relationships can be very helpful in teaching others about cultural sensitivity.

CRITICAL THINKING EXERCISES
1.   Your patient is from a different country and speaks minimal English. Your translator has been to see the patient and has gone over the hospital routines, rules, and list of patient's rights. The patient's mother insists on staying in the room 24 hours a day. She refuses to let you perform assessments and cares on the patient. The patient is in pain, but the mother does not allow pain medication to be given. The patient will not accept the food from the hospital. You smell food cooking and enter the room to find the mother cooking on a hot plate, which is a fire code violation. How can you help this situation?
2.   You are home one evening and you hear the 18-month-old child of your upstairs neighbors. The child has been crying for 3 hours. You have heard no footsteps in the apartment. The answering machine picks up each time you call. You become concerned and call the building supervisor to open the door to the neighbor's apartment. When the supervisor lets you in, you find unsanitary conditions and realize that the parents are not

in the apartment. You look outside and see the parents several apartments down, partying with friends. What are your responsibilities? How will you respond to the parents? Whom would you notify? The parents tell you to "Mind your own business." What will you say to them? What will you do if it happens again?

3. List three situations that were very uncomfortable for you. What defense mechanisms did you use? How could you respond to each of these situations in a more effective manner? List three situations in which you observed someone else using defense mechanisms. How can you help them to cope in a more effective manner?

SAMPLE QUESTIONS

1. The concepts of space, time, and waiting are:

    A. Religious

    B. Cultural

    C. Economic

    D. Ethnic

2. The condition of judging a person or situation before all the facts are known is called:

    A. Hatred

    B. Abuse

    C. Prejudice

    D. Stereotype

ANSWERS AND RATIONALES

1. Answer: B

    Rationale: Space, time, and waiting are cultural concepts. They have different meanings for different people. There are different religions and ethnic groups within cultures. Economic concerns would not directly relate to proxemics from a nursing standpoint.

2. Answer: C

    Rationale: Prejudice is prejudging before knowing all of the facts. Hatred and stereotype may be partially at fault. Abuse may be an outcome of prejudice.

ACTIVITIES

1. Have your students interview a person who is from a different religion or a culture than his or her own. Use the Interview Skill Sheet format from Chapter 7 if you like. Have the student present the results orally or in writing. This will reinforce the information presented in Chapter 7, as well as provide firsthand information pertinent to this chapter.

2. Have the students dress in traditional clothing for their religion or culture. Make the class an *event*—have traditional ethnic foods, music, games, and so on.

3. Many licensed practical nurses/licensed vocational nurses work in the home care field. It is often necessary for the nurse to help the patient with nutrition. The nurse may have

difficulty getting the patient to comply with eating and may label the patient as having a behavior problem when the real problem may simply be differences in what the nurse and patient consider appropriate food. Divide your class into groups of three or four. Assign them a simulated patient from a specific culture that is not common to your geographic area. Each group must design a 1-day menu (breakfast, lunch, and dinner) for that individual, according to the patient's cultural likes and needs. The menu must also comply with a budget that is appropriate for that patient's socioeconomic group. Have the students describe the patient's menu and its approximate cost.

SUPPORTIVE MATERIALS

1.   "Basic Differences" (videocassette), Insight Media, 121 W. 85th Street, New York, NY 10024.
2.   "A Place to Come Back to" (videocassette, 1987), Seraphim Communications, 1568 Eustis Street, St. Paul, MN 55108.
3.   "Parent Perspectives: Raising Children with Emotional Disorders" (videocassette, 1991), PACER Center, 4826 Chicago Avenue So., Minneapolis, MN 55417.
4.   "When Mental Illness Invades the Minority Family" (videocassette, 1991), Alliance for the Mentally Ill/Alabama, 3322 Memorial Parkway #215F, Huntsville, AL 35801.

REFERENCES

Baumrind, D. (1971). Current paterns of paternal authority. *Developmental Psychology* (monograph 1), *4*, 1–103).

Eron, L.D., and Peterson, R.A., "Abnormal Behavior: Social Approaches" Annu. Rev. of Psych. (Rosenzweig, M.R. and Porter, L.W. 1982 p. 231.)

Galanti, G. (1991). *Caring for Patients from Different Cultures: Case Studies From American Hospitals*. Philadelphia: University of Pennsylvania Press.

Merriam-Webster Dictionary. (1994). Springfield, MA: Merriam-Webster, Inc.

Chapter 6

LEARNING OBJECTIVES
1.   Define coping.
2.   Differentiate between effective and ineffective coping.
3.   Define defense (coping) mechanisms.
4.   Identify main defense mechanisms.

KEY TERMS
- Coping
- Defense mechanisms
- Effective coping
- Ineffective coping

Coping
Coping is the way people psychologically adapt to a stressor. It is the ability people develop to consciously deal with problems and stress. Individuals have different methods of coping or dealing with their stressors.

Effective coping skills are those that are specifically identified to offer healthy choices to the patient.

Ineffective coping differs from effective coping in that, when the conscious techniques people try are unsuccessful, they often unconsciously allow themselves to fall into habits that give the illusion of coping. These habits are called **defense mechanisms** (or coping or mental mechanisms) and they are discussed in the following section.

Defense Mechanisms
The purpose of defense mechanisms is to reduce or eliminate anxiety. Surprisingly, when used in very small doses, they can be helpful. Some commonly used defense mechanisms follow in Table 6–1.

Table 6–1   DEFENSE MECHANISMS

MECHANISM	DESCRIPTION	EXAMPLES	OVERUSE CAN LEAD TO:
DENIAL	• Usually the first defense learned and used. • Unconscious refusal to see reality. • Is *not* conscious lying.	The alcoholic states, "I can quit any time I want to."	Repression and dissociative disorders.
REPRESSION (STUFFING)	• An unconscious 'burying" or "forgetting" mechanism. • Excludes or withholds unbearable events/situations from our consciousness. • A step deeper than denial.	"Forgetting" a loved one's birthday after a fight.	

MECHANISM	DESCRIPTION	EXAMPLES	OVERUSE CAN LEAD TO:
DISSOCIATION	• Painful events or situations are separated or dissociated from the conscious mind. • Patients often say, "I had an out-of-body experience," or "It happened to someone else, but it was as though it happened to me."	• Patients who have been sexually abused as a child may describe the situation as if it happened to friends or siblings. • Police officers visit parents to inform them of their child's death in a car accident. Parent tells police, "That's impossible. My child is upstairs asleep. You must have the wrong house."	One of the dissociative disorders, such as multiple personality disorder.
RATIONALIZING	• Use of a logical excuse to cover up true thoughts and feelings. • The most frequently used defense mechanism.	• "I did not make a medication error; I followed the doctor's order." • "I failed the test because the teacher wrote bad questions."	Self-deception.
COMPENSATION	Making up for something perceived as an inadequacy by developing a desirable trait.	• The small boy who wants to be a basketball center becomes an honor roll student instead. • The physically unattractive person who wants to model becomes a famous designer instead.	
REACTION FORMATION (OVERCOMPEN-SATION)	Similar to compensation, except the person usually develops the *exact opposite* trait.	• The small boy who wants to be a basketball center may become a political voice to decrease the emphasis on sports in elementary schools. • The physically unattractive person who wants to be a model may speak out about the elimination of beauty pageants.	Failure to resolve internal conflicts.

MECHANISM	DESCRIPTION	EXAMPLES	OVERUSE CAN LEAD TO:
REGRESSION	• Emotionally returning to an earlier time in life when there was much less stress. • Commonly seen in patients who are hospitalized. *Note*: Not everyone goes back to the same developmental age. This is highly individualized.	• Children who are toilet trained begin wetting themselves. • Adults who start crying and have a "temper tantrum."	• Interference with perception of reality. • Interference with personality development and progression.
SUBLIMATION	Unacceptable traits are diverted into acceptable traits ("socially acceptable").	• Burglar teaches home safety classes. • Person who is potentially physically abusive becomes professional sports figure. • People who choose not to have children run a day care.	Reinforcement of negative tendencies, causing the person to show signs of the undesirable behavior or trait.
PROJECTION (SCAPEGOATING)	• Blaming others, or a mental or verbal finger-pointing at someone else for personal problems.	• "I didn't get the promotion because you don't like me." • "I'm overweight because you make me nervous."	• Finding faults in everything and everyone. • Failure to learn personal responsibility. • Development of delusional tendencies.
Displacement (Transference)	The "kick the dog syndrome." Transferring anger and hostility to another person or object, which is perceived to be less powerful than you are.	Parent loses job without notice; goes home, and verbally abuses spouse; spouse unjustly punishes child; child slaps the dog.	• Loss of friends and relationships. • Confusion in communication.
RESTITUTION (UNDOING)	• Makes amends for a behavior one thinks is unacceptable. • Makes an attempt at reducing guilt.	• Giving a treat to a child who is being punished for a wrongdoing. • The person who sees someone lose a wallet does not return it but puts extra in the collection plate at the next church service.	A double message that relieves the "doer" of the responsibility to of honesty in the situation.
ISOLATION	Emotion that is separated or isolated from the original thought.	"I wasn't really angry; just a little upset."	Avoids dealing with true feeling; can increase stress.
CONVERSION REACTION	Anxiety is channeled into physical symptoms. *Note*: Often, the symptoms disappear soon after the threat is over.	Nausea develops the night before a major exam, causing the person to miss it. Nausea may disappear soon after the exam is over.	Physical disorders, such as gastric ulcers and possibly some types of cancer.

MECHANISM	DESCRIPTION	EXAMPLES	OVERUSE CAN LEAD TO:
AVOIDANCE	Unconsciously staying away from events or situations that might lead to feelings of aggression or anxiety.	"I can't go to the class reunion tonight. I'm just so tired that I have to sleep."	

KEY CONCEPTS

1. Stress and people's responses to it are very individualized. People are not all stressed by the same things, nor they deal with stress in the same way.

2. Defense mechanisms are believed to be a part of the ego from Freud's description of personality. These mechanisms are based, for the most part, in the unconscious, but can appear to be very deliberate.

3. Use of defense mechanisms for a short period of time can be helpful. The mechanisms act as a pressure valve and allow the psyche to put the stress into perspective. If the patient deals with the problem successfully, the outcome can be an effective coping technique; if not successful, the patient's anxiety may increase.

CRITICAL THINKING EXERCISES

1. Phil is a middle-aged male who is brought to your medical unit with possible alcohol poisoning. Phil is in and out of consciousness. He has an IV in his arm for hydration. Phil's wife has just arrived and is asking you, Phil's nurse, about his condition. Phil awakens and sees you speaking with his wife. He simultaneously pulls out his IV and shouts, "Get me out of here. I am fine. I don't need to be in this place. Get me out!"

   Have the student perform a critical evaluation of this situation. What emotions or defense mechanisms might Phil be experiencing? What might be some of his physical responses to the alcohol consumption? What symptoms overlap? As the nurse, what North American Nursing Diagnosis Association (NANDA) diagnosis (relating to Phil's mental health) would the students consider the most appropriate? Have the students provide support for their answers to these questions.

ACTIVITIES

1. In class or as an assignment, have the students write down details of a situation that made them feel very uncomfortable. Then, have them write down how they handled it and if they were satisfied with the outcome of the way they handled it. Next, have them identify the defense mechanisms they may have used to handle the situation. Finally, have the students identify what they will do differently if they are ever in a similar situation.

2. Have the students do the same activity except have them chronicle someone else's uncomfortable situation. It can be a family member, friend, classmate, or anyone else they choose (teachers are exempt, of course). Ask the students if it was easier to do the activity on themselves or other people, and what the rationale is for their choices.

SAMPLE QUESTIONS

1. A person who always sounds like he or she is making excuses is displaying:

   A. Denial

   B. Fantasy

C.   Rationalization

D.   Transference

2.   The alcoholic who says, "I don't have a problem. I can quit any time I want to; I just don't want to," is displaying:

   A.   Denial

   B.   Fantasy

   C.   Dissociation

   D.   Transference

3.   Your young male patient tells you that he may not be big enough for the basketball team, but "that's alright because I'm a 4.0 student and I'm on the principal's list." Your patient is displaying:

   A.   Denial

   B.   Transference

   C.   Dissociation

   D.   Compensation

MATCHING QUESTIONS
Directions
Match the defense mechanism in column A with the example in column B. On the answer sheet, write the letter of the response from column B next to the corresponding number of column A. Use each response only once; there is an extra response.

Column A
1.   Compensation
2.   Repression
3.   Regression
4.   Denial
5.   Conversion
6.   Projection/scapegoating
7.   Dissociation
8.   Fantasy

Column B
A.   Painful ideas/feelings/events separated from awareness
B.   A believable false story
C.   Also called escapism
D.   Retreat to earlier, less stressful time
E.   "I can quit drinking any time I want to."
F.   "I'm overweight because you make me so nervous I have to eat."
G.   "I might be too short for basketball but I'm great in music!"
H.   Anxiety that is channeled into physical symptoms
I.   Stuffing of painful thoughts/feelings

ANSWERS AND RATIONALES
Sample Questions
1.   Answer: C

Rationale: Rationalization is the defense mechanism that makes that person sound like he or she is always making excuses.

2.   Answer: A

Rationale: Denial is the refusal to accept situations for what they really are. This is a classic example of denial.

3.   Answer: D

Rationale: This patient is using compensation. Compensation is finding a strength that makes up for a real or imagined inadequacy.

Matching
1.   G.
2.   I.
3.   D.   To "regress" means to go "backward."
4.   E.   Failure to accept behaviors or situations as they truly are.
5.   H.   Anxiety that is "converted" from emotional symptoms into physical symptoms.
6.   F.   Pointing the "blame" at another takes the responsibility from the individual and projects it on the other person.
7.   A.   Emotional pain that is too severe for the individual to endure is divorced or dissociated from the conscious memory.
8.   C.   As a defense mechanism, this is a form of escaping mental trauma. *Caution*: fantasy can be used consciously in some forms of therapy.

REFERENCES
    Bailey, D.S., and Bailey, D.R. (1993). *Therapeutic Approaches to the Care of the Mentally Ill*, 3rd ed. Philadelphia: F.A. Davis.
    Barry, P.D. (1994). *Mental Health and Mental Illness*, 5th ed. Philadelphia: J.B. Lippincott.
    Bauer, B.B., and Hill, S.S. (1986). *Essentials of Mental Health-Care Planning and Interventions*. Philadelphia: W.B. Saunders.
    Crawford, A.L., and Kilander, V.C. (1985). *Psychiatric and Mental Health Nursing*, 6th ed. Philadelphia, F.A. Davis.
    Kalman, N., and Waughfield, C.G. (1993). *Mental Health Concepts*, 3rd ed. Albany, NY: Delmar Publishers.

LEARNING OBJECTIVES
1.   Define the role of the LPN/LVN in the five steps of the nursing process.
2.   State need for nursing process in mental health issues.
3.   State concepts of patient interviewing.
4.   Prepare a patient interview.
5.   Collaborate in creating a nursing process for a given patient.
6.   State concepts of patient teaching.
7.   Prepare and implement a teaching exercise.

KEY TERMS
- APNA
- Data collection
- Evaluation
- NANDA
- Nursing diagnosis
- Nursing process
- Implementation
- Patient teaching
- Plan of care

Note to Teacher: Included at the end of this chapter is a form you may copy or adapt to use in having your students practice the Nursing Process from a Mental Health rather than a Medical-Surgical emphasis. There are also four hypothetical case studies to accompany the Nursing Process project. Suggested grading is also included on the form.

STEP 1: ASSESSING THE PATIENT'S MENTAL HEALTH
The role of the licensed practical nurse/licensed vocational nurse (LPN/LVN) in this first step of the **nursing process** is to *assist* with assessment.

Interviewing Techniques
For purposes of this text, the word "interview" pertains to any nurse-patient interaction that requires the nurse to obtain specific information from the patient. The interview is usually the primary method of data-gathering used in health care (Anderson, 1990). It is important to collect data about the whole person. Data related to thoughts and feelings are as important to any nurse-patient interview as the physical data the nurse collects.

Intake/Admission Interview
It is up to the nurse to rephrase the questions in an open-ended format that seems more personalized to the patient.

> **EXAMPLE:**
> Standard forms probably say, "Married? _____YES _____NO."
> Nurse interviewer can ask, "What is your marital status?"
>
> OR
>
> Standard form: "Do you smoke or use alcohol? ____YES _____NO."
> Nurse interviewer: "How often do you smoke or use alcohol?"

Helping Interview

The helping interview is used to determine or isolate a particular concern of the patient and to help the patient to learn to help himself or herself.

Guidelines for Nurse-Patient Interviewing

1. *Be honest.* Tell the patient the purpose of the interview.
2. *Be assertive.* If the interview is mandatory (intake, preoperative, and so on), the patient must understand that this is required. Contract for a mutually acceptable time to do the interview so the patient will be prepared.
3. *Be sensitive.* Sometimes the questions are very difficult or embarrassing for the patient to answer. Assure the patient that you understand his or her feelings and that the information you are given is part of his or her medical record. Only the patient, the patient's designee, and people who are involved in his or her caregiving will have access to this information.
4. *Use empathy.* Let the patient know that you are interested in what is being said and that you are there to be helpful. Acknowledge the patient's feelings but do not judge them.
5. *Use open-ended questions.* Personalize the questions as much as possible. Use this time to discuss and clarify as much information as you can in order to avoid having to repeat parts of the interview later.

Note to Teacher:

The following is a form for "interviewing" that you may copy or use as a guide to meet your needs. Suggested grading points are also included.

Interview Skill Grading Sheet

This interview skill is designed to be a hands-on exercise to help learn to develop and execute an effective interview that can be used in future nursing-related interviews. You will be graded in the three following areas: use of the APIE process format, style and quality of questions/communication techniques, and time factor.

Suggested Grading

1. **APIE Format**

_____ Assessment statement (1 point possible)

_____ Plan statement (1 point possible)

_____ Implementation (5 points possible)

_____ Evaluation statement (1 point possible)

2. **Style and Quality of Questions**

_____ Relevant to assessment and goal of interview (4 points possible)

_____ Open-ended questions (4 points possible)

_____ Nonverbal communication affects verbal communication (4 points possible)

3. **Time Factor**

_____ (5 minutes allowed, at 1 point per minute = 5 points possible)

STEP 2: DEFINING PATIENT PROBLEMS

Processing the data that has been collected is a function of the registered nurse (RN), according to the American Nurses' Association (ANA). The American Psychiatric Nurses Association (**APNA**) has published a set of nursing diagnoses specific to psychiatric disorders. It is the RN's responsibility to assimilate the data that have been collected and choose one or more potential nursing diagnoses for the patient.

STEP 3: PLANNING CARE

The LPN/LVN role is again a partner in care planning. The ANA believes that the RN has the primary responsibility for this step of the nursing process. Planning care involves setting of short- and long-term goals from the patient's perspective, not from the nurse's perspective.

STEP 4: IMPLEMENTATIONS/INTERVENTIONS

The LPN's role is to assist with identifying and carrying out the specific steps that will help the patient reach set goals. Nurses are able to provide input about new interventions that may be helpful, but the LPN is the person who begins to help adapt certain procedures to assist the patient. Nurses also need to understand the rationale the implementations that are selected and be prepared to explain them to patients and the patients' families.

Many of the implementations or interventions that are helpful to the patient involve **patient teaching**.

Everyone needs a little help to get started teaching, regardless of what sort of teaching will be done.

Teaching in any form is most effective when it is started as soon as possible after admission. Nurses teach patients in different ways. Teaching falls under the categories of either formal teaching or informal teaching. Formal teaching is any situation in which there is a class scheduled or specific objective that must be met. Informal teaching, or adjunctive teaching, happens anytime and anywhere the patient is in need of information.

Nurse-teachers need to have a basic understanding of the principles of teaching and learning. Some of these principles follow.

Principles of Learning
1. Each person learns differently.
2. Each person learns at his or her own pace.
3. People learn best when the information is *meaningful* to them.
4. Learning is most effective when the information is presented in small segments.
5. *Success breeds success.*

Principles of Teaching
1. *Know your patients.*
2. *Know your material.*
3. *Have a teaching plan.* A very simple format such as the APIE format for the nursing process can be adapted for teaching, as follows:

   A= Assessment. What is the need for the teaching? Who are the patients? How much time is available? Assessing for the need to teach can be as simple as one or two statements. For example, "Good afternoon, everyone. My name is Sandy. This is the class on colostomy care and it is open to anyone with a colostomy and their significant others."

   P= Plan. In true nursing process, this is often called the goal. What do you plan to accomplish in the session? How do you think you will do it? Again, this can be accomplished in one or two statements. For example, "This is the first in a series of three classes and the task for today is to learn about the different types of appliances and equipment you have available to you."

I= Implementation. This is the step-by-step method you will perform in order to accomplish the plan. It is similar to the implementation portion of the nursing process. You will have as many or as few steps as you need. There will, however, be critical items that you will need to cover with all patients to meet legal and safety issues.

E= Evaluation. In a teaching plan, you evaluate the patient's learning, as well as your own performance. How do you know that the patient has grasped the concepts and skills from the class? What do you look for? Do you need to ask for a return demonstration? Does it need to be perfect? How did you do? Did you achieve the plan? Did you have enough time? Too much time? What will you do differently next time? How did your students evaluate the session? Your evaluation criteria may change from time to time as well.

4. *Be flexible.*
5. *Be able to evaluate the learning.* In health teaching in the facility, this can be in the form of a question-answer session, a short quiz, or a return demonstration.
6. *Plan to stay a few minutes after the class for questions.* Even though you may ask for and welcome questions during the session, there are always people who are not comfortable asking questions in a group. They will want your time in private, so allow some time to either clarify their concern at the time or to set up a time to help later in the day.
    The typical methods used in health teaching are lecture and demonstration.
1. *Lecture.* This is a method that is designed for information giving. It is very unilateral; the nurse talks, the patients listen. Lecture classes may include videos, slides, or charts.
    Evaluation of student learning from the lecture method is traditionally assessed by quizzes or question-answer sessions. Because not all patient participants are comfortable answering in a group, it may be difficult to assess how much learning each individual has achieved.
2. *Demonstration.* Demonstration is an excellent technique to follow an introductory lecture. For visual and tactile learners, it is a preferred method of learning.
    Demonstrations are effective because, after the initial demonstration, the nurse-teacher can go around to each individual and give one-on-one help or redemonstration. Evaluation for the method of teaching is usually the redemonstration.
3. *Be honest.* Nobody said a nurse must have all of the answers. If you do not know something, admit it. Go look it up and either bring the information to the individual who asked, or bring it to the next session of the class.
4. *Have fun!* Teaching can be a very rewarding part of nursing. There is no better way to reinforce your own knowledge than to teach it to someone else. It is one way of being generative and keeping the nursing culture alive.

STEP 5: EVALUATING INTERVENTIONS
This final step of the nursing process is also one in which the LPN/LVN plays an assisting role.

KEY CONCEPTS
1. Nursing process is an example of collaborative nursing practice. RNs are primarily responsible for the steps of the nursing process; LPN/LVN-prepared nurses assist in data collection, planning, implementing, and evaluating the nursing process.
2. Nurses are performing more interviewing and teaching on a daily basis. Entry-level nurses need to have a basic knowledge of both of these skills. The nurse's state and facility sets the guidelines of teaching within the scope of practice.
3. Nursing process is a helpful tool for preparing a teaching plan.
4. The ANA has set guidelines that dictate the roles of the RN and the LPN/LVN in collaborating in the nursing process.

CRITICAL THINKING EXERCISES

1. Your state Nurse Practice Act allows you, the LPN/LVN, to oversee care and function as a charge nurse, as long as an RN is on call. Your medical patient has gone out on a 3-hour pass with relatives and returns to your agency refusing to perform the interventions as stated on the care plan. Your patient is argumentative but answers questions appropriately. Your data collection includes fruity odor on breath, mood swings, and hunger. You need to make some corrections or additions to the care plan, but are unable to make contact with the RN on call. What do you think might be considered as nursing diagnoses? What interventions can you perform and still remain within your state's scope of nursing practice?

2. Assist in preparing a nursing process. With the information given within the nursing process scenarios, complete steps of the nursing process as requested. The instructor may have more examples. There can be more than one solution.

3. Pick a student partner to interview. Pick any topic. Develop a 5-minute interview. Write it twice: once with only closed-ended questions and aggressive statements and once with only open-ended questions and assertive statements. Compare the two versions. How was it different as the interviewer and how was it different for the interviewee?

4. Pick a topic to teach the class. This can be any topic you are comfortable with. You have 10 minutes (classroom instructor may choose own time limit) to teach your topic. Develop a teaching plan. Teach your topic. Evaluate your teaching. What would you do differently the next time?

SAMPLE QUESTIONS

1. The nursing process is a method for:

   A. Systematic organization and implementation of patient care

   B. Documenting patient needs

   C. Differentiating RN role from LPN/LVN role

   D. Data collection

2. You are assisting in collecting data on a new patient in your unit. The physician suspects alcohol abuse. You want to find out the patient's history and frequency of alcohol use. Your best choice for collecting this data might be:

   A. "Do you use alcohol?"

   B. "How often do you get drunk?"

   C. "How many times a week would you say you drink alcohol?"

   D. "Why do you use alcohol? It's bad for you."

3. When doing patient teaching, the best method to evaluate the success of the patient is:

   A. Lecture

   B. Redemonstration

C.   Implementation

D.   Assessment

4.   The mental status exam is done in what part of the nursing process?

A.   Assessment

B.   Plan

C.   Implementation

D.   Evaluation

ANSWERS AND RATIONALES

1.   Answer: A

Rationale: Nursing Process is a systematic way of collecting data to have consistency in patient care. Options B and C are incorrect, even though nurses do document patient needs and RN and LPN/LVN roles are different in the nursing process. Patient needs are not usually documented as part of the nursing process per se. Option D is incorrect because the nurse needs to know the difference between medical and nursing care prior to writing the nursing process. Only nursing care is incorporated into the nursing process.

2.   Answer: C

Rationale: This is the best choice of those listed. It asks what you need to know but asks from the patient's perspective. It is less judgmental than the other choices.

3.   Answer: B

Rationale: Return demonstration (redemonstration) is the best method for evaluating the patient's learning. Option A is a method of teaching. Options C and D are steps in the nursing process and steps in developing a teaching plan.

4.   Answer: A

Rationale: Mental status examinations are done as part of the assessment or data collection part of the nursing process.

REFERENCES

Anderson, C. (1990). *Patient Teaching and Communicating in an Information Age.* Albany, NY: Delmar Publishers.

Hill, S.S., and Howlett, H.A. (1993). *Success in Practical Nursing—Personal and Vocational Issues*, 2nd ed. Philadelphia: W.B. Saunders.

Note to Teacher: There are two forms included for your use. One form is for single teaching and the other is for team teaching. The criteria are slightly different but it gives you the option to allow for class size, time limits, and so on. You may copy these or use them as a guideline to write to your own needs. It is helpful to assign points and include this in your grading system. These forms also allow you to grade on spelling and grammar, as well as the other content.

SINGLE TEACHING

1. Pick a topic—nursing related is preferred, but can be anything the student is comfortable with.
2. Plan for 10 minutes; time is crucial for nurses!
3. Complete teaching plan.
4. Hand in the completed teaching plan as you finish your teaching.
5. If you need something from your instructor, please request it in writing at a time of the instructor's choosing.

TEAM TEACHING (COLLABORATIVE EXERCISE)

1. Sign up in pairs.
2. Pick a topic—nursing related is preferred, but can be anything that the team is comfortable with.
3. Plan for 15 minutes; time is crucial for nurses!
4. Complete teaching plan. Work is to be mutually agreed upon as being equally distributed. This is a collaborative project.
5. Contract for the amount of points you are working for if your instructor has assigned points.
6. Hand in the completed teaching plan as you finish your teaching.
7. If you need something from your instructor, please request it in writing at a time of the instructor's choosing.

TEACHING PLAN

Name: _____

Names (if team teaching): _____

_____

Topic: _____

Time started: _____ Time stopped: _____ Time used: _____

Assessment:

Plan:

Implementation:

Evaluation:

Suggested grading (possible total 10 points)

Assessment: 0–2

Plan: 0–2

Implementation: 0–2

Evaluation: 0–2

Time: 0–2

(10 minutes for single teaching; 15 minutes for team teaching)

Team teaching only: We are contracting for _____ points. We have agreed that the foregoing expectations were completed and that the work was equally distributed.

Points earned: _____

NURSING PROCESS PAPER

Student Name: _____

DIRECTIONS: You will get a case study. You will have *minimal* information about the patient in the case study. Treat the case study as if the patient was in your clinic and you were compiling information to collaborate with the RN in charge. From the information presented in your case study, write your nursing process paper. Use a separate sheet of paper. There will be information enough to fill in all of the blanks below. There is more than one right solution to the case study.

I.   Social history (2 points)
II.   Medical history (past/present [2 points])
III.   Describe the behavior you see (4 points)
IV.   Define previous behaviors in nursing diagnosis terms (must be *complete* nursing diagnosis [2 points])
V.   Write a care plan for the two previous nursing diagnoses (10 points)

I. PROBLEM   GOAL   NURSING INTERVENTIONS

                                    1.

                                    2.

                                    3.

                                    4.

                                    5.

II. PROBLEM   GOAL   NURSING INTERVENTIONS

                                      1.

                                    2.

                                    3.

                                    4.

                                    5.

VI.   Describe *your feelings* about caring for a patient showing this behavior. How will you need to adapt or change your communication skills in order to be therapeutic for this patient? (5 points)

     Two or more spelling/documentation errors (-1 point)
     (*Total* 25 points)

Note to Teacher: There are three examples of case studies which you may use as the given data collection for your LPN/LVN students as they practice the nursing process from a mental health standpoint. Remember that there is purposely minimal information in these case studies. The setup should include instructions that the patient may be unwilling or unable to give information, and the nurse is to do the best with what information is there. The nurse is also expected to find ways to obtain information. You may give as much or as little guidance as your state designates to the RN role.

CASE STUDY #1: Mrs. Penn

Mrs. Penn, age 44, is admitted to the hospital for diagnostic studies. Her physician suspects peptic ulcer as the cause of her symptoms. At the time of her admission, Mrs. Penn appears pale, underweight, and in generally poor health. Diagnostic tests ordered by her physician include a complete blood count, gastric analysis, and an upper gastrointestinal series.

The evening before the gastric analysis is scheduled, you tell Mrs. Penn that in preparation for the x-ray, she is not allowed to eat or drink anything after midnight. She becomes very apprehensive and tells you that she has never heard of a gastrointestinal series. She asks what they will do to her when she gets her x-ray and why she has to have the test.

Mrs. Penn tells you that she has recently been divorced from an alcoholic husband and she wonders if the emotional upsets she has suffered have any bearing on her present physical condition.

Mrs. Penn's physician initially decided to treat the ulcer medically. He ordered a bland diet and Maalox every other hour. Because of continued tension in Mrs. Penn's daily life and her obvious inability to stay within the limits of her diet, even in the hospital, the physician has now decided to perform a subtotal gastrectomy, vagotomy, and jejunostomy. Prior to her surgery, a nasogastric tube was inserted and gastric decompression was accomplished by attaching the tube to suction.

CASE STUDY #2: The Bicks

Mr. Bick, age 70, suffers from chronic obstructive lung disease, or chronic obstructive pulmonary disease (COLD/COPD). He has had asthma for years and smoked one and one-half to two packs of cigarettes daily. He has also had shortness of breath on exertion for many years, but recently has begun to experience occasional bouts of dyspnea, even when at rest. His most recent admission to the hospital is for treatment of an acute respiratory infection, which have made his symptoms more severe. He has an almost constant cough that is essentially nonproductive.

Mrs. Bick wishes to be of some help during her husband's recent illness. She asks many questions and seems to understand what is happening. She is concerned about the disposal of the nasal and bronchial secretions and prevention of infection to herself and others. She states that she "knows of people who have developed tuberculosis" in similar circumstances.

Mr. Bick's physician orders intermittent positive-pressure breathing (IPPB) therapy four times daily after the acute infection subsides. The physician also orders physical therapy to start Mr. Bick on exercises that will improve his respiratory function. Mr. Bick returns from physical therapy quite short of breath and wants to have oxygen for an hour afterward.

After a week of treatment, the physician tells the Bicks that Mr. Bick no longer needs acute care, and will discharge Mr. Bick today or tomorrow. The nurse requests the social services department to come and talk with the Bicks because Mrs. Bick has refused to take him home "while he is still so sick."

CASE STUDY #3: A.H.

A.H. is a 40-year-old patient admitted to your floor from the emergency department. A.H. is a native of another country, where English is not the primary language; however, the medical record indicates that A.H. speaks English. The patient has been in the United States for 3 years and works in the hospitality industry. A.H. has had a minor stroke; physical symptoms are reduced, but A.H. does not allow any physical cares to be performed. Nurses work hard to convince A.H. to allow them to complete vitals and neurological checks. A.H. does not eat and does not take the medications ordered by the physician. Family arrives, but A.H. still does not permit care to be given.

Note to Teacher: Following is a form you may copy or adapt to have your students practice the nursing process from a mental health rather than a medical-surgical emphasis.

CLINICAL ACTIVITY

1.   If your students are at a point in their curriculum that places them in clinical care, assign this activity for one of the clinical experiences. Have them complete a simple mental status exam on one of their medical-surgical patients. They must address all eight areas of the exam in some way:
   - Level of awareness/orientation
   - Appearance and behavior
   - Speech/communication
   - Affect
   - Thinking
   - Perception
   - Memory
   - Judgment
2.   If you can, and if your clinical affiliates will allow, arrange for students to follow with a nurse from the mental health unit. Have the student write a summary of the experience, including observations of communication, rapport, patient responses, and so on.

Chapter 8

LEARNING OBJECTIVES
1.   Describe a therapeutic milieu.
2.   Identify classifications, uses, actions, side effects, and nursing, as well as considerations for four classifications of psychoactive medications.
3.   Describe psychoanalysis.
4.   Describe behavior modification.
5.   Describe rational emotive therapy.
6.   Describe humanistic/person-centered therapy.
7.   Identify nurse's role in counseling.
8.   Describe three types of counseling.
9.   Describe concepts of group therapy.
10.   Describe electroconvulsive therapy (ECT) and nurse's role in ECT.
11.   Define crisis.
12.   Identify the five phases of crisis and nurse's role in them.

KEY TERMS
- Antidepressants
- Antimanic agents
- Antipsychotics
- Behavior modification
- Cognitive
- Counseling
- Crisis
- ECT
- Hypnosis
- Milieu
- Person-centered
- Psychopharmacology
- Psychoanalysis
- Rational emotive

Milieu
(*Note to teacher:* I have left this area blank, so that you can customize your own discussion of this topic.)

Psychopharmacology
(*Note to teacher:* I have left this area blank, so that you can customize your own discussion of this topic.)

Antipsychotics
Extrapyramidal side effects of medications (EPS): These are serious side effects and must be observed for very carefully. They are as follows:
1.   Parkinsonism
2.   Akathisia
3.   Dystonia
4.   Tardive dyskinesia

Some examples of antipsychotic medications are chlorpromazine hydrochloride (Thorazine), haloperidol (Haldol), trifluoperazine hydrochloride (Stelazine), and fluphenazine enanthate (Prolixin Enanthate).

Antianxiety Agents
Common antianxiety agents are alprazolam (Xanax), buspirone hydrochloride (Buspar), diazepam (Valium), propanolol hydrochloride (Inderal), and lorazepam (Ativan).

Antidepressants
(*Note to teacher:* I have left this area blank, so that you can customize your own discussion of this topic.)

Antimanic Agents
(*Note to teacher:* I have left this area blank, so that you can customize your own discussion of this topic.)

Psychotherapies
The goals of psychotherapy are to:
1. Decrease the patient's emotional discomfort
2. Increase the patient's social functioning
3. Increase the patient's ability to behave or perform in a manner appropriate to the situation

Psychoanalysis
Some of the techniques used in psychotherapy are:
- Free association
- Dream analysis
- Hypnosis/hypnotherapy
- Catharsis
- Behavior modification

Cognitive Therapies
- Rational emotive therapy
- Person-centered/humanistic

Counseling
- Group therapy
- **Electroconvulsive therapy (ECT)**

Crisis Intervention
Most experts categorize crisis into five stages, or phases. The following table outlines the five phases of crisis and the behaviors that are often seen during those phases.

Table 8–1   THE FIVE PHASES OF CRISIS

PHASE	BEHAVIORS
PRECRISIS	Person feels "fine". Will often deny stress level, and, in fact, state a feeling of well-being.
IMPACT	Person feels anxiety and confusion. May have trouble organizing personal life. Stress level is high. Person will acknowledge feeling stress but may diminish its severity.

PHASE	BEHAVIORS
CRISIS	Person denies problem is out of control. Withdraws or rationalizes behaviors and stress. Frequently uses defense mechanism of projection. (May last varied amounts of time.)
ADAPTIVE	Person perceives crisis in a positive way. Anxiety decreases. Person attempts to regain self-esteem and is able to start socializing again. Is able to do some positive problem solving.
POSTCRISIS	Surprisingly, both positive and negative functioning may be seen. Person may have developed a more positive, effective way of coping with stress *or* may show ineffective adaptation, such as being critical, hostile, depressed, or may use food or chemicals, such as alcohol, to deal with what has happened.

Goals of Crisis Intervention

The goals of crisis intervention change according to the degree of treatment you are involved in. In any case, the first goal of any crisis intervention is to take care of the immediate or precipitating problem. Other goals of crisis intervention are as follows:

1. Ensure safety
2. Diffuse the situation
3. Determine the problem
4. Decrease anxiety level
5. Return patient to precrisis (or better) level of functioning

Legal Considerations

It is always safer for nurses to do something. Exactly what nurses are able to do depends greatly on their locale, level of preparation, state's Nurse Practice Act, and comfort level.

Patients have a choice of either voluntary treatment commitment or involuntary commitment.

KEY CONCEPTS

1. The place where treatment is given must be conducive to therapy. "Milieu" is the word used to describe the environment of the treatment area.
2. Psychopharmacolgy is very important to the effective treatment of patients. There are many classifications of psychoactive medications and many individual medications within each of these classifications. It is the nurse's responsibility to consult a drug reference regarding all psychotropic medications that they give to patients. It is also part of the nurse's role to reinforce teaching about the medications to the patient.
3. Psychotherapy is used to treat patients. Sometimes, it is used in conjunction with medications. There are several methods of psychotherapy, such as psychoanalysis, behavior modification, rational emotive therapy, and humanistic/person-centered therapy.
4. Counseling is carried out in different ways, depending on the patient's needs and the type of illness. Counseling may be licensed and regulated differently from state to state and municipality to municipality. A nurse's role in counseling varies accordingly with these regulations. Counseling is carried out individually or in group settings, according to the situation.
5. ECT is used for specific situations. Premedication is usually ordered. It is the role of the nurse to monitor vital signs, maintain safety, and document posttreatment observations.

6. Crisis intervention is very individualized. There are five phases of crisis and each person experiences them differently.

CRITICAL THINKING EXERCISES

1. With a student partner, role-play one or more of the following potential crises (or think up your own). Think about your communication techniques. Do they change when dealing with crisis? If so, how? What about your nonverbal communication techniques?
   - Parent whose child has been abducted at the mall
   - Man who calls the clinic states that he has just killed his wife
   - Woman who is frantically seeking shelter from an abusive relationship
   - Adolescent friend of your child who slashes his or her wrists as you are talking; you are home alone
   - Alcoholic, who is the main wage earner for the family, has just been fired from job

SAMPLE QUESTIONS

1. Which of the following is *not* a behavior noted in the *crisis* phase of crisis?

   A. Denial

   B. Feeling of well-being

   C. Use of projection

   D. Rationalization

2. One of the first statements a nurse might make to a person in crisis is:

   A. "Why didn't you leave the first time you were attacked?"

   B. "Do you want to prosecute or not?"

   C. "What do you think made him or her hit you?"

   D. "You're safe here, and I would like to help you."

3. A therapeutic environment (milieu) is *best* defined as:

   A. An environment in which a patient is under a 72-hour hold

   B. An environment that is locked and supervised

   C. An environment that is structured to decrease stress and encourage learning new behavior

   D. An environment that is designed to be homelike for persons who are hospitalized for life

4. Which of the following does *not* state a goal of psychotherapy?

A. Decrease emotional pain/discomfort

B. Increase social functioning

C. Increase ability to behave appropriately

D. Allow patient to avoid/deny uncomfortable situations

5. Which of the following is *false* regarding electroconvulsive therapy (ECT)?

A. It is used to treat depression and schizophrenia.

B. It is used to stop convulsive seizures.

C. Fatigue and disorientation are immediate side effects.

D. Memory will gradually return.

6. Psychopharmacology (psychotropic drug therapy) is used:

A. As a cure for mental illness

B. Only to control violent behavior

C. To alter the pain receptors in the brain

D. To decrease symptoms and facilitate other therapies

7. Mrs. Henderson has been started on chlorpromazine hydrochloride (Thorazine). As her nurse, you are teaching her about the possible side effects of this antipsychotic drug. Which of the following will you include in your teaching?

A. Photosensitivity

B. Weight loss

C. Elevated BP

D. Hypoglycemia

8. Avoiding such foods as bananas, cheese, and yogurt should be stressed to patients who are taking:

A. Fluoxetine hydrochloride (Prozac)

B. Lithium carbonate

C. Monoamine oxidase inhibitors (MAOIs)

D. Tricyclic antidepressants

9. The goals of crisis intervention include all of the following *except*:

A. Safety

B. Increasing anxiety

C. Taking care of the precipitating event

D. Return to precrisis or better level of functioning

10. In order for psychotherapy to be effective, it is necessary to do all of the following *except*:

A. Encourage the patient to repress feelings

B. Reinforce appropriate behavior

C. Establish a therapeutic patient-staff relationship

D. Assist patient to gain insight into problem.

11. When forming a nursing diagnosis for a mental illness/behavior problem, you should:

A. Look only at physical symptoms

B. Focus on psychological needs and include physical needs

C. Realize that goals will be met quickly

D. Evaluate the plan

12. Mr. Douglas is being treated with haloperidol (Haldol, an antipsychotic) for organic dementia. He is at first hard to arouse, then stays sleepy after the next three doses. You know sedation may occur with this drug. As his nurse, your first nursing action would be:

A. Notify your supervisor; call the physician

B. Realize that tolerance will occur and continue giving the drug

C. Immediately discontinue the drug

D. Administer an antidote

13. It is 8 days later. You enter Mr. Douglas' room and observe tremors of his face and hands, drooling, and flat affect. You are probably observing signs of:

A. Acute dystonia

B. Parkinsonism

C. Acute drug toxicty

D. Withdrawal

14. If an EPS such as tardive dyskinesia occurs, the treatment of choice is to:

A.   Administer anticholinergic drugs, as ordered

B.   Discontinue the drugs per order

C.   Increase the dose per order

D.   Administer antianxiety drugs per order

15.   Your patient, Mrs. L is on your unit for bowel resection. She is exhibiting signs of nervousness and anxiety, which she attributes to the upcoming surgery. You note from her record that she has a history of ethyl alcohol (ETOH) abuse. Which of the following classifications of drugs would be potentially addictive for her?

A.   Lithium salts

B.   Antianxiety drugs

C.   Antipsychotic drugs

D.   Anticholinergics

ANSWERS AND RATIONALES

1.   Answer: B

Rationale: Options A, C, and D are commonly seen in the *crisis* (or third) phase of crisis. A feeling of well-being is observed in the *precrisis* phase of crisis, when the patient thinks and states that everything is "fine."

2.   Answer: D

Rationale: The patient needs to know that he or she is away from the stress, even if it is only temporary. The patient may not be able to think rationally, and to hear that safety and help are being offered can be the start of stress reduction and intervention. Option A is wrong because the word "why" needs to be avoided when possible to decrease the chance of the statement sounding judgmental and allowing the patient to feel defensive. Option B is a closed-ended question and the person may not know the answer. It may, in fact, be one of the major causes of the stress that led to the crisis. Option C is an open-ended statement and will be valid to ask at a later time. As one of the first questions a person in crisis hears, it can lead to increased confusion and guilt.

3.   Answer: C

Rationale: Milieu is the therapeutic environment. It should be stress free, or at least minimally stress producing and should make the patients feel comfortable to practice new, healthy behaviors. It might be locked, depending on the patients, but it is not required to be. The patients are not usually hospitalized "for life" (some might be, though) and a 72-hour hold situation will have a milieu that corresponds to the needs of the patient being held.

4.   Answer: D

Rationale: Avoidance and denial are some targets for treatment with psychotherapy, not goals of psychotherapy. Options A, B, and C are all goals of psychotherapy.

5.   Answer: B

Rationale: ECT is not used to treat convulsive disorders. That is a mistake people make because of the name "electroconvulsive therapy." The treatment causes a light seizure but does not treat seizure disorders.

6.   Answer: D

Rationale: Using psychoactive medications can change the person's ability to think and process information and can help he or she feel differently about the situation, which may allow other therapies to work in adjunct with the medication, to help the person toward wellness. These medications do not cure mental illness. They are used for more than just violent behavior and, though they may have an effect on pain receptors, that is a side effect, not a primary use for this group of medications.

7.   Answer: A

Rationale: Photosensitivity is a frequent side effect of this group of medications, especially chlorpromazine hydrochloride (Thorazine). Patients need to understand that they can burn easily out in the sun and should take precautions to stay shaded or keep their skin covered.

8.   Answer: C

Rationale: Patients taking MAOIs should avoid certain foods that may cause them to go into hypertensive crisis; these are foods contain tyramine.

9.   Answer: B

Rationale: One of the goals of crisis intervention is to decrease anxiety. The person may feel a temporary increase in anxiety (e.g., at the time of being arrested or taken to the detox center), but that should resolve fairly quickly with effective intervention.

10.   Answer: A

Rationale: Repression is a defense mechanism and is therefore counterproductive in therapy.

11.   Answer: B

Rationale: Mental health nursing is a holistic practice. These nurses take care of the whole person, not just the mind or the body. Treatment in many cases is not achieved quickly and may involve lifelong work on the part of the patient. Evaluating the plan is another part of the nursing process. Option A is incorrect because it is the nurse's responsibility to notify the supervisor and to call the physician according to scope of practice. The remaining choices are not independent nursing functions.

12.   Answer: B

Rationale: These are symptoms of the EPS of parkinsonism.

13.   Answer: A

Rationale: Anticholinergics are the usual drugs of choice for decreasing the effects of EPS.

14.   Answer: B

Rationale: The antianxiety drugs are potentially addictive. A person with addictive tendencies may become addicted to these medications more easily than other medications.

ACTIVITY
1.   Plan time at the end of your class period to play a tape or video of a crisis situation; however, do *not* let the students know the outcome of the crisis and do *not* plan enough time for discussion until the next class. (This might be as hard on you as it is on your students, but it is very effective.) Have students note:
   - The problem
   - The response of the person intervening
   - Communication skills
   - What they *feel* about the situation
   - What they would do differently

Then, send them away until the next class period. Do not answer any questions about the outcome of the crisis until then. (I have found that your law enforcement/9-1-1 agency may release actual calls for you to use during this activity. The name of the caller will need to be erased for confidentiality). Can you think of other crisis situations to use for this activity?

2.   Choose several of the primary diseases and have your students research and present them. Three to four students per group seems to divide the work nicely. A technique that works well is to choose one specific disease from a group for the students to present, and then you present the other illnesses from that group (e.g., students present paranoid schizophrenia, you lecture on the disorganized and catatonic types).

        This project will teach research, organization, written communication, and collaboration, as well as the disease. It will involve some effort on your part because each group is to write two multiple choice questions that will be incorporated into their next exam. The questions and answers should be written on the exam exactly as the students have worded them, but you may change the order of the answer options (so they do not all memorize the answers. A sample form follows, which you may copy for your own use.

3.   Work with the hospital where you do your clinical rotations. Try to assign each student a clinical day or part of a clinical day in the emergency room. The student should observe for examples of crisis or mental health issues. Each student should complete a set of objectives and report to the clinical group in your postconference time.

GROUP PRESENTATION FOR MENTAL HEALTH ALTERATIONS

Directions

Your instructor will choose a disease for your group to present. This is a group project with a group grade. The group will collaborate on the project and will contract for the grade they are working for. You will complete this form and present it to the instructor as part of the grade.

Criteria

Each presentation will be a minimum of one-half hour long. Each group will present the signs, symptoms, medical care and nursing interventions for that disease. Each group will write two multiple-choice questions that will be incorporated into the next examination. Your instructor will give you specific direction for this.

GROUP LEADER: _____ DISEASE: _____

GROUP MEMBERS: _____

_____

GRADE CONTACTING FOR: _____

PLAN FOR REACHING THIS GRADE: (TEACHING PLAN): _____

_____

_____

_____

TEST QUESTION #1 (WITH ANSWER OPTIONS):

_____

_____

A. _____ C. _____

B. _____ D. _____

TEST QUESTION #2 (WITH ANSWER OPTIONS):

_____

_____

A. _____ C. _____

B. _____ D. _____

DID YOU MEET YOUR CONTRACT AGREEMENT? _____

IN WHAT WAYS?

_____

_____

DATE PRESENTED_____

POINTS/GRADE GRANTED_____

Special Credit:
Johnson, J., 9-1-1 Dispatch Program, Minneapolis Technical College Minneapolis, 1996.

SAMPLE OBJECTIVES
1.   Identify the crisis or mental health situations(s) you observed. Do *not* use patient names or other identifiers, please.
2.   List the signs and symptoms (i.e., behaviors, physical appearance, and so on.) to support the crisis or mental health situation you observed.
3.   Who was assigned to care for this person?
4.   What forms of communication were used (include examples of verbal and nonverbal communication)? What was the patient's response to the communication?
5.   Instructor may add other objectives as appropriate.

SUPPORTIVE MATERIALS

1.   "A Guide to Rational Living" with Dr. Albert Ellis (videocassette, 1988), from the series "Thinking Allowed," 5966 Zinn Drive, Oakland, CA 94611.
2.   "Succeeding With Imaging and Self-Hypnosis-Exercises in Personal Growth" (audiocassette, 1993), Dr. Allen R. Zimmerman, Communi-Care Inc., 20550 Lake Ridge Dr., Prior Lake, MN 55372. FAX: 612-492-5888

LEARNING OBJECTIVES
1.   Define anxiety disorders.
2.   Identify five specific anxiety disorders.
3.   State physical and behavioral symptoms of five anxiety disorders.
4.   Identify treatment modalities for five anxiety disorders.
5.   Identify nursing care for five anxiety disorders.

KEY TERMS
- Anxiety
- Compulsion
- Eustress
- Free-floating anxiety
- Generalized anxiety
- Obsession
- Panic disorder
- Phobia
- Post-traumatic stress
- Signal anxiety
- Stress
- Stressor

Stress is everywhere in our society. Stress from positive experiences is called **eustress**. It can produce just as much anxiety as the negative stressors. A **stressor** is any person or situation that produces anxiety responses. **Anxiety** is the uncomfortable feeling of dread that is a response to extreme or prolonged periods of stress. It is rated as mild, moderate, severe, or panic (Kalman and Waughfield, 1993).

Anxiety may also be influenced by one's culture. Anxiety is usually referred to in two ways: (1) **free-floating anxiety**, which is described as a feeling of impending doom, and (2) **signal anxiety**, which is an uncomfortable response to a known stressor.

Differential Diagnosis
Symptoms of anxiety disorders can mimic those seen in diabetes, cardiac problems, medication side effects, electrolyte imbalances, or physical trauma. The physician needs to rule out a systemic infection or an allergy.

Types
Generalized Anxiety Disorder (GAD)
In GAD, the anxiety itself is the expressed symptom. Symptoms may include:
- Muscle aches
- Shakes
- Palpitations
- Dry mouth
- Nausea
- Vomiting
- Hot flashes
- Chills
- Polyuria
- Trouble swallowing

Panic Disorder

Panic is a state of extreme fear that cannot be controlled. Some of the behaviors that may be observed in **panic disorder** include:

- Fear (usually of dying, losing control of self, or of "going crazy")
- Dissociation (a feeling that it is happening to someone else or not happening at all)
- Nausea
- Diaphoresis
- Chest pain
- Increased pulse
- Shaking
- Unsteadiness

Phobia

Phobia is defined as an irrational fear and is the most common anxiety disorder.

Psychoanalytic view implies that it is really not the object that is the source of the fear but a fear of the defense mechanism displacement.

There are three subcategories of phobias: agoraphobia, social phobia, and simple phobia. Agoraphobia is the irrational fear of being someplace and being unable to leave or being very embarrassed if leaving is required. Social phobias are those in which people avoid social situations due to fear of humiliation. Simple phobia is an irrational fear of a specific object or situation. This phobia is the one we hear most about. Examples of simple phobias are claustrophobia (fear of enclosed places), hematophobia (fear of blood), and acrophobia (fear of heights).

Obsessive-Compulsive Disorder (OCD)

OCD is a different type of anxiety disorder that consists of two parts: the **obsession** (repetitive thought, urge, or emotion) and the **compulsion** (repetitive act that may appear purposeful). The thought or the action is the mechanism that reduces the anxiety.

Defense mechanisms that have been associated as possible contributors to OCD are repression, reaction formation, and undoing.

Behaviors are varied. Each person performs the thought or action that is the substitute for the anxiety-producer. Some people wash their hands unceasingly. Others have a strict ritual that, if it is interrupted, requires starting over from the beginning. Some people have to check something or clean something over and over. People with this disorder tend to be perfectionists and very rule oriented.

Physical symptoms also vary. If the person is prevented from performing the obsession or compulsion, the anxiety converts itself into somatic (body-related) symptoms.

Post-Traumatic Stress Disorder (PTSD)

PTSD is developed in response to some unexpected emotional or physical trauma that the person could not control. War, rape, violent storms, or violent acts are possible causes of this trauma.

A term associated with PTSD is "survivor guilt." Survivor guilt is the feeling of guilt expressed by those who "made it" through a traumatic event. Symptoms include:

- "Flashbacks," in which the person may relive and act out the traumatic event
- Social withdrawal
- Feelings of low self-esteem as a result of the event
- Relationships with significant others may change and new relationships may be difficult to form
- Irritability and outbursts of anger toward someone or some situation occur, seemingly for no obvious reason obvious
- Depression

- Chemical dependency may occur as a physical or behavioral response to the traumatic experience

Medical Treatment for People with Anxiety Disorders

Treatment is individualized for the patient. Psychopharmacology usually involves the antianxiety classification of medications. Individuals with anxiety disorders who are chemically dependent are managed with other medications that are not primarily used for the treatment of anxiety disorders, but that may have calming qualities. Examples of these drugs are hydroxyzine hydrochloride (Atarax), clonidine hydrochloride (Catapres), and sertraline hydrochloride (Zoloft). (Shives, 1994). Antidepressants and antipsychotics are also effective for some people. If these medications arc not effective in treating the symptoms, monoamine oxidase inhibitors (MAOIs) or lithium carbonate may be prescribed.

Counseling is individually suited to the patient.

Nursing Interventions for People with Anxiety Disorders

1. Maintain a calm milieu
2. Maintain open communication
3. Observe for signs of suicidal thoughts
4. Document any behavioral changes
5. Encourage activities

KEY CONCEPTS

1. Anxiety disorders have many common characteristics. There are psychoanalytic theories that hold the belief that it is important to find the underlying cause of the anxiety. Biologic theories believe that the causes are not the primary concern, but rather the physical reasons that may result in the anxiety.
2. Medications and therapies are individualized for the patient.
3. Trust and communication techniques are important tools for the nurse caring for a patient who has an anxiety disorder. Maintaining a calm milieu is also essential.

CRITICAL THINKING EXERCISES

1. Tommy has come to your clinic with numerous cracks on his hands. They are bleeding and very sore. Tommy tells you that he just has to wash his hands all the time. His mother says he washes for 2 to 3 hours at a time, and he does not stop when she tells him to. The physician has diagnosed Tommy with OCD and has explained the illness to Tommy and his mother. When the physician leaves the room, Tommy's mother begins to cry and says, "What did he just say? What am I supposed to do? What did I do wrong that Tommy got this illness?" What will you tell her? What areas will you explore with her?
2. Jeanne is a 21-year-old single woman who is admitted for pneumonia. Her social history indicates that she survived a house fire when she was 10-years-old, though her twin sister died in that fire. Today is the day for the hospital's monthly fire drill. You note that Jeanne is not in her bed. You are unable to find her during the drill. After the drill, you search her room and find her sitting on the floor of the closet. She is wrapped in a blanket and is crying. She does not respond to your verbal cues. What do you think is happening to her? What illness might she have? How will you get her out of the closet? What can you do to help her?
3. Your 13-year-old child has been having episodes of nausea, diarrhea, and malaise. He or she denies having trouble with friends or school, saying, "I just don't feel good, Mom. Can I please stay home? Please?" On parent-teacher meeting day, however, you find out that the episodes of illness are directly related to major exams. When you confront your

child, he or she denies any correlation. What do you think is happening? What can you do to help? How will you help your child help himself or herself?

SAMPLE QUESTIONS

1. Your significant other is a veteran of the Gulf War. It is very difficult for him or her to drive through a parking ramp because "there are people hiding behind the pillars! They have guns! Be careful!" This person is most likely experiencing:

   A. Auditory hallucinations

   B. Flashbacks

   C. Delusions of grandeur

   D. Free-floating anxiety

2. The previous situation indicates what type of anxiety disorder?

   A. Generalized anxiety disorder (GAD)

   B. Phobia

   C. Post-traumatic stress disorder (PTSD)

   D. Obsessive-compulsive disorder (OCD)

3. Mrs. T cannot leave her home without checking the coffeepot numerous times. This makes her late to many functions, and she occasionally misses engagements because of it. Mrs. T is probably suffering from what kind of anxiety disorder?

   A. GAD

   B. Phobia

   C. PTSD

   D. OCD

4. Mr. L has a severe fear of needles. He is hospitalized on your medical unit. The lab technician enters to draw blood for the routine complete blood count (CBC) and Mr. L cries out, "Get away from me! I can't breathe! I'm having a heart attack!" Your first response to Mr. L would be:

   A. "I'll take your vital signs and call my supervisor."

   B. "Why do you think you're having a heart attack, Mr. L?"

   C. "Don't worry. She's done this many times before."

   D. "Relax, Mr. L. Take a few deep breaths. I'll stay with you."

5. Which of the following is *not* an anxiety disorder?

A. Panic disorder

B. OCD

C. Multiple personality disorder

D. PTSD

6. Mr. Uneasy states, "I never feel at ease. I always have a feeling of dread. I just know something is going to go wrong." He is experiencing:

A. Signal anxiety

B. Free-floating anxiety

C. Test anxiety

D. Atypical anxiety

7. A patient with OCD is:

A. Suspicious and hostile

B. Flexible and adaptable to change

C. Extremely frightened of something

D. Rigid in thought and inflexible with routines and rituals

8. Which of the following is *true* regarding a phobic disorder?

A. It involves a repetitive action.

B. It involves a loss of identity.

C. It results in sociopathic behavior.

D. It is an irrational fear that is not changed by logic.

9. Nursing interventions for anxiety disorders include all of the following *except*:

A. Encouraging the patient to verbalize thoughts and feelings

B. Informing the patient of expected behaviors and consequences

C. Withholding information from the patient to lessen stress

D. Allowing the patient to control as much of his or her care as possible

10. In OCD, a compulsion is a

A. Repetitive thought

B. Repetitive action

C.   Repetitive fear

D.   Repetitive illusion

ANSWERS AND RATIONALES

1.   Answer: B

Rationale: The vividness of the description suggests that the person is having a flashback. Auditory hallucinations would most likely involve "voices" or "hearing" the guns. Delusions of grandeur might cause the person to go after the people with guns while being unarmed himself or herself. Free-floating anxiety would be less descriptive. The person would not know the cause of the anxiety.

2.   Answer: C

Rationale: The behaviors indicate the probability of PTSD.

3.   Answer: D

Rationale: The repetitive behavior that interferes with daily functioning is indicative of OCD.

4.   Answer: D

Rationale: This is the best choice because you are simply stating for the patient to relax, helping him reoxygenate and refocus, and calming him by offering to stay with him. It also buys you some time to make a visual assessment. Option A would be appropriate nursing actions, but not as the first priority. Your first action needs to be calming the patient and continuing to assess. B and C are nontherapeutic responses.

5.   Answer: C

Rationale: Multiple personality disorder, or dissociative identity disorder, is considered to be a dissociative disorder rather than an anxiety disorder. Some theorists say that the dissociative disorders are also anxiety disorders, but most theorists are now differentiating between the two disorders.

6.   Answer: B

Rationale: The feeling of impending doom is characteristic of free-floating anxiety. Signal anxiety is an anxiety response to expected events, such as tests.

7.   Answer: D

Rationale: Rigid and inflexible behaviors are characteristic of OCD. People would like to control these behaviors, but it is very difficult without treatment. They are not usually hostile unless they are prevented from performing the obsession or compulsion, because that *is* what decreases the anxiety.

8.   Answer: D

Rationale: A phobia is an irrational fear that cannot be changed by reason or logic. The patient usually understands it is irrational, but the fear remains.

9. Answer: C

Rationale: Withholding information that the nurse thinks might cause stress is not a helpful action for the patient. If the physician has not already informed the patient, or if the nurse states his or her discomfort about discussing the information, that is another consideration, but arbitrarily deciding to withhold information from the patient may actually increase the patient's anxiety.

10. Answer: B

Rationale: A compulsion is a repetitive act; an obsession is a repetitive thought.

REFERENCES
Kalman, N., and Waughfield, C.G. (1993). *Mental Health Concepts*, 3rd ed. Albany, NY: Delmar Publishers.
Shives, L.R. (1994). *Basic Concepts of Psychiatric-Mental Health Nursing*, 3rd ed. Philadelphia: J.B. Lippincott.

LEARNING OBJECTIVES
1.   Define mood disorder.
2.   Identify four types of mood disorders.
3.   State physical and behavioral symptoms of four mood disorders.
4.   Identify treatment modalities for four mood disorders.
5.   Identify nursing care for four mood disorders.

KEY TERMS
- Affect
- Bipolar
- Cycle
- Dysthymia
- Hypomania
- Mania
- Mood

Mood disorders (or affective disorders, as they are also referred to) are disorders in which people experience extreme changes in **mood** (emotions) and **affect** (the outward expression of the mood).

Etiologic Theories
Psychoanalytic theory indicates that people who have suffered loss in their life are the ones who will develop depressions.

Cognitive theorists believe that an individual's perception of events may lead to depression.

Biologic theories offer more options as to why people develop depressions. Chemical imbalances and genetic links are two popular ideas. Studies on identical twins also offer different possibilities. Statistics from the National Institutes of Health (NIH) indicate that if one identical twin develops a mood disorder, the other has a 70 percent chance of developing the same disorder.

Approximately twice as many women as men report feeling depressed. Biologic theorists, however, believe that there is a connection between female hormones and the neurochemicals. Some of the general symptoms that frequently occur are low or depressed mood, flat affect, sleep disturbances, constipation, irritability (especially in children and adolescents), fluctuations in weight (in either direction), and withdrawal from usual friends and activities.

Differential Diagnosis
Symptoms of depression may occur as a result of other disorders, such as schizophrenia and drug side effects or overuse. Symptoms can mimic congestive heart failure, nutritional deficiencies, fluid and electrolyte imbalances, infections, or diabetes.

Types
Major Depression (Unipolar Depression)
People who develop major depression exhibit a vast array of symptoms. These symptoms may be the same behaviors everyone displays as they progress through the "normal" ups and downs of life. People who have major depression just show them more strongly and for a greater period of time than those who are not clinically depressed. Behavioral and physical symptoms include:
- Sad mood

- Loss of pleasure in usually pleasurable things
- No hallucinations or delusions and four of the following for at least 2 consecutive weeks:
  - Weight loss or gain resulting from increased or decreased appetite
  - Sleep pattern disturbances
  - Increased fatigue
  - Increased agitation
  - Increase or decrease in normal activity; lowered pleasure for life, including sexual activity
  - Feelings of guilt or worthlessness
  - Decreased ability to think, remember, or concentrate
  - Suicidal thoughts

Dysthymic Depression (Dysthymia)

Dysthymia is defined as severe depression for a period of at least 2 years for adults and at least 1 year for adolescents and younger children. Symptoms of dysthymia include:

- Low or depressed mood that lasts the greater part of every day for the 2-year period
- According to *Diagnostic and Statistical Manual of Mental Disorders* (Fourth Edition) (*DSM-IV*), at least two of the following:
  - Overeating or undereating
  - Insomnia or hypersomnia
  - Low energy or fatigue
  - Low self-esteem
  - Poor ability to make decisions
  - Feelings of hopelessness
  - Anhedonia (inability to feel pleasure)
- *DSM-IV* states that at least three of the following must be present:
  - Low energy levels
  - Altered sleep patterns (either more or less than usual)
  - Feelings of worthlessness and sadness
  - Pessimism about the future
  - Psychomotor slowing
  - Recurring suicidal thoughts
  - Loss of pleasure in activities that were once pleasurable

Bipolar Depression

Bipolar depression (manic depressive illness, or bipolar disorder, as it is also called) is the type of depression in which both extreme **mania** (extreme elation or extreme agitation) and extreme depression exist. It only takes one episode of mania to actually be diagnosed with bipolar disorder, but it is more common to see the patient alternate or **cycle** from one "pole" to the other.

Hypomania is a term used to describe behavior that is similar to that of mania but not as severe.

The U.S. Department of Health and Human Services, Alcohol, Drug Abuse and Mental Health Administration (1993) lists the following signs of mania and depression. Signs of mania are as follows:

- Excessive highs or feelings of euphoria
- Sustained period of behavior that is different from usual
- Increased energy, activity, restlessness, racing thoughts, and rapid talking
- Decreased need for sleep
- Unrealistic beliefs in one's abilities and powers
- Extreme irritability and distractibility
- Uncharacteristically poor judgment
- Increased sexual drive
- Abuse of drugs, particularly cocaine, alcohol, and sleeping medications
- Obnoxious, provocative, or intrusive behavior

- Denial that anything is wrong

Signs of depression are as follows:
- Persistent sad, anxious, or empty mood
- Feelings of hopelessness or pessimism
- Feelings of guilt, worthlessness, or hopelessness
- Loss of interest or pleasure in ordinary activities, including sex
- Decreased energy, a feeling of fatigue or being slowed down
- Difficulty concentrating, remembering, and making decisions
- Restlessness or irritability
- Sleep disturbances
- Loss of appetite and weight loss or gain
- Chronic pain or other persistent bodily symptoms that are not caused by physical disease
- Thoughts of death or suicide; suicide attempts

DSM-IV agrees with these symptoms, but adds that symptoms must be present for specified periods of time, depending on the type of depression (NIH, 1993).

Involutional Depression/Melancholia

Involutional depression or melancholia generally affects people over age 45. It, too, seems to affect women more frequently than men and has been nicknamed "empty nest syndrome" because symptoms generally appear or become pronounced after the last child leaves home. Symptoms are more somatic than other types of depression. Anorexia and sleep disturbances are common. Hypochondriasis may occur.

Medical Treatment for People with Depressive Disorders

Depression often goes untreated; one in three people with depression actually seek treatment. With treatment, approximately 80 percent of people with serious depression can be helped in a matter of a few weeks. (NIH, 1994).

Lithium carbonate is the drug of choice, in most instances, for the treatment of bipolar depression. Antidepressants may also be used.

Psychotherapy for the patient and family may also be used. Play therapy is the most frequent and effective form of therapy for children.

Electroconvulsive therapy is an option when other forms of therapy are not effective.

Nursing Interventions for People with Depressive Disorders
1. Patience, patience, patience!
2. Monitor lithium levels. (Normal range of lithium is 1.0 to 1.5 mEq/L while loading and 0.6 to 1.2 mEq/L when on maintenance.)
3. Honesty
4. Consistency
5. Activity
6. Nutrition
7. Communication

KEY CONCEPTS
1. Depressive disorders are common threats to mental health in the American population.
2. Signs and symptoms of depressive disorders are similar to the behaviors common in all people who experience the usual ups and downs of daily life.
3. It is often the degree of severity and length of time that the symptoms are present that determines whether the person is clinically depressed or what type of depression is present.

4.   Some forms of depressive disorders are easier to treat than others. Patients may need to be on medications for long periods or perhaps for the rest of their life. People who develop melancholia may never improve.

CRITICAL THINKING QUESTIONS

1.   You are one of the team of school nurses in a local high school. You notice that Maria, a 17-year-old student, is behaving oddly. She has always been rather loud and has even been referred to as "obnoxious" by several of her peers. Lately, you have observed her sitting alone, as if waiting for someone, but, when you approach her, she barely greets you and then leaves. What are your concerns about Maria? What are some of the possibilities that might be affecting her? How will you approach her more effectively the next time you see her?

2.   Your sister-in-law calls you at home one day to talk about your brother. You have all been concerned about Marcus since he lost his job last year. He has been unable to find adequate employment. Your sister-in-law has had to get two part-time jobs so that Marcus can continue to interview. He has been in a very low mood, has quit the bowling team and has been sleeping 10 to 12 hours daily. Today, however, your sister-in-law is excited. "Marcus is a new man! I don't know what happened, but he just got a burst of energy. He told me not to worry about a thing because he was first in line for the position of president at the local bank. He said I could quit my job! He went out and bought a new car. Isn't that great?" What should you think about your brother? What questions should you ask your sister-in-law? What actions will you take when you talk to Marcus?

SAMPLE QUESTIONS

1.   You admit Mr. N to your unit. He is a 49-year-old male who is pleasant and compliant. He admits to being "a little down. My last son left for college 1000 miles away. I feel so empty, especially since his mother died last year." The physician ordered fluoxetine hydrochloride (Prozac) for Mr. N, but you observe no change in his behavior, and on a scale of 1 to 5, Mr. N describes his mood as "somewhere below that 5." You suspect Mr. N is suffering from what type of depressive disorder?

   A.   Major depression

   B.   Bipolar depression

   C.   Dysthymic disorder

   D.   Melancholia

2.   Ms. S is admitted to your medical unit with a diagnosis of dehydration and a history of depression. She tells you, "I just can't eat. I'm not hungry." Your best therapeutic response would be:

   A.   "You aren't hungry?"

   B.   "If you can't eat, what is that candy bar wrapper doing in your bed?"

   C.   "Why aren't you hungry?"

   D.   "You really should try to eat some real food."

3. Janey, a 7-year-old child, is hospitalized in your unit for treatment of depression. Among other forms of treatment, you would expect to be involved in what type of therapy with Janey?

    A. Rational emotive

    B. Play

    C. Transactional analysis

    D. Work

4. Mrs. Outofsync is admitted to your medical-surgical unit with a diagnosis of dehydration and pneumonia. She has a history of bipolar disorder, which is controlled by medication. As her nurse, you know you must:

    A. Treat her carefully because she may become catatonic

    B. Observe for signs of lithium toxicity from dehydration

    C. Alert the other staff members of the "psycho" on the unit

    D. Treat the medical illness only

5. Mr. Quiet is describing the fire that destroyed his home 2 weeks ago. His wife and son were critically injured and they lost all of their material possessions. He has burns over 70 percent of his body. His voice is dull, and he has no change in facial expression. This *outward display* of emotion is called:

    A. Ambivalence

    B. Flight of ideas

    C. Mood

    D. Affect

6. To communicate well with Mr. Quiet, you do all of the following *except*:

    A. Develop a trust

    B. Show acceptance

    C. Be judgmental

    D. Be honest

7. Mr. Quiet tells you he feels responsible for his family's injuries and does not know if he can face them. He states, "I think it would be better if I died." After leaving his room, your next action(s) is/are:

A. Document the conversation, inform the charge nurse and the physician, and observe the patient

B. Document the conversation but omit the part about him dying, because he probably did not mean it

C. Keep the information to yourself because it is confidential

D. Tell his wife so that she can reassure him.

8. From the previous information, which of the following is the best problem/focus to use in forming a nursing diagnosis for Mr. Quiet?

A. Noncompliance

B. Manipulation

C. Ritualistic behavior

D. Guilt

9. The nurse who is assessing a patient with major depression (unipolar depression) would expect to observe which of the following symptoms?

A. Euphoria

B. Extreme fear

C. Extreme sadness

D. Positive thinking

10. The nursing interventions for this patient with major depression would include all of the following *except*:

A. Active listening skills

B. Maintaining a safe milieu

C. Encouraging adequate nutrition

D. Reassuring the patient that everything will be "just fine"

ANSWERS AND RATIONALES

1. Answer: D

   Rationale: Men, as well as women, can suffer from this type of "empty nest syndrome." His symptoms are not consistent with the other depressive disorders and the fact that his medication does not help him may be a clue that this is a harder form of depression to treat, although it has only been a short treatment time.

2. Answer: A

Rationale: This is selective reflecting. You have repeated the patient's exact words in a way that encourages her to either explain herself or rephrase her response. Options B, C, and D are all blocks to therapeutic communication. B challenges her, C uses the word "why," and D gives advice.

3. Answer: B

Rationale: Play therapy is the most common and most effective form of therapy for children. Work (or occupational) kinds of therapy, behavior modification, and rational emotive therapy are a little far advanced for a child of this age.

4. Answer: B

Rationale: Lithium is an electrolyte. Dehydration could increase the chances of lithium's severe side effects.

5. Answer: D

Rationale: Affect is the outward display or physical display of an emotion.

6. Answer: C

Rationale: Communicating in a judgmental manner is always a block to therapeutic or helping relationships.

7. Answer: A

Rationale: Documenting the interaction, informing the charge nurse and the physician, and observing the patient are the best nursing actions at this time. Omitting part of the conversation is not appropriate. Maintaining patient confidentiality is required.

8. Answer: D

Rationale: From the patient's comments about feeling responsible for the plight of his family, guilt would be the best choice. Manipulation sounds plausible, but people in this condition are generally not trying to deliberately manipulate others.

9. Answer: C

Rationale: Major depression usually manifests with symptoms of extreme sadness that has been the prevalent mood for a period of 2 years. Euphoria would be more indicative of bipolar depression.

10. Answer: D

Rationale: This is the block of false reassurance, which is never appropriate in therapeutic relationships. The other choices are all appropriate nursing interventions for a person who is depressed.

ACTIVITY
1. Have the students write in a journal about their moods. Determine the time frame for the journal. Students should write in the journal at least once daily (including weekends). (This number should increase, as they should write in their journals each time they notice

their moods changing.) They should identify the mood, describe the situation surrounding the mood change, offer suggestions as to why the situation affected their mood, and describe what they did about the mood (i.e., become angry, confront the mood, and so on.) Journals may be collected for grading *or* students may write a summary of their journal that may also be collected for grading.

SUPPORTIVE MATERIALS
1. "Mood Disorders" (videocassette, 1992), from the series, The World of Abnormal Psychology, Annenberg/CPB Collection P.O. Box 2345, S. Burlington, VT 05407-2345.
2. "Depression" (vidcocassctte), from the series Health Talk and U University of Minnesota Media Resources, Rarig Center, 330-21st Avenue So. Minneapolis, MN 55455
3. "Taking Control of Depression" (videocassette, 1991), Xenejenex, 300 Brickstone Square, Andover, MA 01810.

REFERENCES
Hendrix, M.L. (1993). *Bipolar Disorder—Decade of the Brain*. (NIH Pub. No. 93-3679). (Formerly DHHS Publication No. (ADM) 90-1609. Washington, DC: Alcohol, Drug Abuse and Mental Health Administration).

McEnany, G. (1990, September). Managing mood disorders. *RN, 53*, 28.

National Institutes of Health. (1994). *Helpful Facts About Depressive Illnesses*. (DHHS-NIH Pub. No. 94-3875). Bethesda, MD: National Institutes of Health.

LEARNING OBJECTIVES
1.   Define personality.
2.   Identify seven types of personality disorders.
3.   State physical and behavioral symptoms of seven personality disorders.
4.   Identify treatment modalities for people with personality disorders.
5.   Identify nursing care for people with personality disorders.

KEY TERMS
- Personality

Webster defines **personality** as "...2. The collection of emotional and behavioral traits that characterize a person; 3. Distinction of personal and social traits..." (Merriam-Webster, 1994). Personalities include thoughts, feelings, and attitudes.

A personality disorder is considered to be a maladaptive behavior, resulting from ineffective personality development.

Etiologic Theories
Most of the major theorists believe that personality disorders originate in early childhood.

The biologic theorists and geneticists are not quite in agreement with the behaviorists and psychoanalytic theorists, however. Again, largely because of tests done on identical twins, it is strongly suggested that if one twin has a personality disorder, the other twin is very likely to have the *same* disorder (Kaplan and Sadock, 1985).

Types
Borderline Personality Disorder
Borderline personality disorder (BPD) is quite common. It is seen more frequently in females. People who display BPD display erratic behavior.

Paranoid Personality
People who have paranoid personality present with behaviors of suspiciousness and mistrust of other people.

Schizoid Personality
People with schizoid personality do not want to be involved in interpersonal or social relationships. They have very few, if any, social interactions, appear to be shy and introverted, have trouble developing friendships with others, tend to respond in a very serious manner that is pleasant, but not warm or inviting.

Dependent Personality
Diagnostic and Statistical Manual of Mental Disorders (Fourth Edition) (*DSM-IV*) defines dependent personality as a "pervasive pattern of dependent and submissive behavior." People with dependent personality want others to make decisions for them, tend to feel inferior and suggestible, have a sense of self-doubt, tend to appear helpless, and avoid responsibility. On the other hand, they tend to take everything to heart and go out of their way to satisfy people they feel close to.

Narcissistic Personality

People with narcissistic personality disorder present behaviors almost opposite of people with schizoid personality disorder. People who have the narcissistic personality tend to display an exaggerated impression of themselves.

Passive-Aggressive Personality
People with passive-aggressive personality disorder present with passive-type behaviors. They arc procrastinators, and they are pouty and irritable. They "forget" to do things they have been asked to do. This disorder, however, seems to be the result of parents who are overbearing and have expectations that are too high for the child to successfully achieve. These parents are probably authoritarian.

Antisocial/Sociopathic Personality
This group of people probably causes the greatest amount of trouble for society. People with this disorder require immediate self-gratification; are often in trouble with the law; have difficulty handling frustration and anger; seldom feel affection, loyalty, guilt, or remorse; and show very little concern for the rights or feelings of anyone else. This group is also at high risk for substance abuse.

It is widely believed that the roots of this disorder relate to parenting and family life. It seems to affect males more frequently than females.

People who have this disorder are usually gregarious, intelligent, and likable. Because of their intelligence, they learn the "jargon" of psychology and know how to manipulate it. They are a difficult to treat.

Medical Treatment for People with Personality Disorders
Medical treatment can be very difficult because patients do not perceive a problem, are very rarely hospitalized for their personality disorders, and often have some misplaced anger that they direct at their therapists. They often leave treatment. Treatment is specifically designed for the patient and may include psychotherapy, individual or group therapy, or cognitive therapy.

Medications may also be used. Fluoxetine (Prozac) is being used with some success.

Nursing Interventions for People with Personality Disorders
The ultimate goal of nursing care for the person who has a personality disorder is increased motivation and socialization. The following are crucial to successful nursing interventions:
1. Unconditional positive regard
2. Trust
3. Limit-setting
4. Communication
5. Role-modeling
6. Safety/security

KEY CONCEPTS
1. Personality disorders are maladaptive responses to personality development.
2. People who have personality disorders are seldom hospitalized for them. They do not see a need for obtaining help and are not always taken seriously by the medical community.
3. When people with personality disorders are brought into treatment, they seldom stay for any length of time; therefore, treatment is rarely successful.

CRITICAL THINKING QUESTIONS
1. You have just admitted Jonathan, a 40-year-old male, to your unit. Jonathan is an executive with a major auditing company. He is being treated for a bleeding gastric ulcer. He is unmarried, 20 lb overweight, and balding. He delights in telling the nursing staff members about his sexual escapades. "Why give all of this magnificence to one person?

No, I'll never commit to a monogamous relationship; not as good a catch as I am!" What personality disorder would you think Jonathan is displaying? How will you converse with him? What limits will you set on his behavior with you?

SAMPLE QUESTIONS

1. When setting limits with patients who have personality disorders, the consequences to those limits should be set:

    A. When the behavior is done

    B. Just before the nurse anticipates the behavior

    C. When the staff or family complains about the behavior

    D. When the limit is set

2. David is a 30-year-old male who comes to your unit for treatment of multiple broken bones following a car accident. He is friendly and flirtatious but very demanding. As you take your data from him, you learn the police are looking for him for petty theft. He laughs and says, "Like they don't have better things to do!" He states that he has changed jobs three times in the past year and has just broken off his second engagement. His former fiancée is visiting and privately tells you that you need to be careful because "he doesn't always tell the truth." You suspect which of the following personality disorders?

    A. Paranoid

    B. Dependent

    C. Antisocial

    D. Schizoid

3. A primary mechanism used by people who have personality disorders is:

    A. Manipulation

    B. Depression

    C. Projection

    D. Euphoria

4. Nurses understand that, for the person with a personality disorder, which of the following behaviors would be the most difficult for the patient to comply with?

    A. Listening to music

    B. Abiding by the hospital's rules

    C. Playing volleyball

    D. Developing a friendship

5.   The person who is in trouble with the law would probably have which of the following personality disorders?

    A.   Narcissistic

    B.   Schizoid

    C.   Antisocial

    D.   Borderline

6.   People who display very erratic behavior most likely have which of the following types of personality disorders?

    A.   Narcissistic

    B.   Schizoid

    C.   Antisocial

    D.   Borderline

7.   Characteristics of paranoid personality disorder include:

    A.   Suspiciousness and mistrust

    B.   Gregariousness and joviality

    C.   Fear and withdrawal

    D.   Hallucinations and seductiveness

8.   Your patient has been admitted with a diagnosis of bilateral pneumonia. You have trouble communicating with this patient, who is pouty and seems to procrastinate and forget to do tasks you have requested. Besides the pneumonia, you ask the physician if there is a history of which of the following personality disorders?

    A.   Schizoid

    B.   Antisocial

    C.   Passive-aggressive

    D.   Borderline

9.   Nursing care for people with personality disorders includes all of the following *except*:

    A.   Unconditional positive regard

    B.   Trust

    C.   Limit-setting

    D.   Vague communication (to decrease feelings of inferiority)

ANSWERS AND RATIONALES

1. Answer: D

   Rationale: Consequences should always be stated when limits are first set. This increases consistency. The following are rationales for the wrong choices: Option A—When the behavior occurs, the patient may be testing, but if the consequences are not known, the patient has not been given enough information to make an appropriate choice. Option B—Anticipating a behavior is presuming and you may be presuming incorrectly. This sets up negative expectations from the patient. Option C—the limits should not be set for the convenience of the staff or family or anyone but the patient. Family should be involved in the care plan only if the patient is agreeable.

2. Answer: C

   Rationale: David is most likely displaying signs of antisocial personality disorder. He does not exhibit signs of suspiciousness or paranoia, and he is not behaving in a dependent manner.

3. Answer: A

   Rationale: Manipulation is used by patients who have personality disorders; however, it is *not* commonly used by patients who have other threats to their mental health.

4. Answer: D

   Rationale: Interpersonal relationships are among the most difficult activities for a person with a personality disorder to develop. They can participate in group activities because they can excel and bring attention and gratification to themselves, but developing a close personal relationship is very difficult.

5. Answer: C

   Rationale: Antisocial (psychopathic) personality is usually the type of disorder in which a person would be in trouble with the law.

6. Answer: D

   Rationale: Erratic behavior is most characteristic of borderline personality.

7. Answer: A

   Rationale: Suspicion and mistrust, especially of other people, are characteristics of paranoid personality disorder. These characteristics are not as serious as they appear when part of paranoid schizophrenia.

8. Answer: C

   Rationale: This patient displays behaviors consistent with passive-aggressive personality disorder.

9. Answer: D

Rationale: Vague communication is not acceptable. Honesty and clarity in communication is always necessary. The patient may feel inferior, which may be part of the manipulation. The nurse needs to confront the feelings or inferiority or any feelings that the patient might state.

ACTIVITY
1.   Have students draw out of a hat one of the personality disorders discussed in the textbook. Have them keep the disorder they have drawn a secret. Have them research the disorder further and, tomorrow, (or next class period or a time of your choosing) come to class in the character of the disorder they researched. The rest of the class should try to identify the disorders being displayed by their classmates.

REFERENCES
Kaplan, H.L., and, Sadock, B.J. (1985). *Modern Synopsis of Comprehensive Textbook of Psychiatry* (4th ed.). Baltimore: Williams and Wilkins.

LEARNING OBJECTIVES
1.   Define schizophrenia.
2.   Identify three types of schizophrenia.
3.   State physical and behavioral symptoms of three types of schizophrenia.
4.   Define the 4 A's of Eugene Bleuler.
5.   Identify treatment modalities for people who have schizophrenia.
6.   Identify nursing care for people who have schizophrenia.

KEY TERMS
- Catatonia
- Delusions
- Hallucinations
- Illusions
- Schizophrenia

The term **schizophrenia** (which means "split mind") was invented by a Swiss psychiatrist, Eugene Bleuler, who used a system of "4 A's" to define schizophrenia. The "4 A's" are:
- Associative disturbance, or looseness
- Affect
- Autism
- Ambivalence

In addition to the "4 A's", patients with schizophrenia display other common symptoms of **delusions**, **hallucinations**, and **illusions**.

Etiologic Theories
Schizophrenia is becoming more widely thought of as a group of illnesses rather than a single condition. Schizophrenia seems to strike adolescents and young adults between the ages of 16 and 25 (Rubin, Peplau, and Salovey, 1993).

There are both psychoanalytic and biologic theories into the causes of schizophrenia.

Differential Diagnosis
It is common for people with schizophrenia to display other thought disorders.

Use of drugs such as mescaline and lysergic acid diethylamide (LSD) can produce behaviors that very closely mimic those seen in patients with schizophrenia. These behaviors are usually short-lived but may produce some permanent damage to the brain.

Types
Paranoid Schizophrenia
The main symptom of paranoid schizophrenia is suspiciousness. In fact, people who have this type of schizophrenia may not exhibit many of the symptoms present in other types.

Patients with this type of schizophrenia tend to have delusions of persecution and grandeur.

Disorganized Schizophrenia
People who have disorganized schizophrenia will display unusual behavior and facial contortions. Speech may be very bizarre and incoherent.

Auditory hallucinations are present but tend to be disorganized.

Catatonic Schizophrenia

Catatonic schizophrenia is seen less frequently than other types, largely due to effective medications. In catatonic schizophrenia, the patient's motor activity is greatly disturbed. People with catatonic schizophrenia vacillate between extreme muscle rigidity and agitation. They sometimes display echolalia/echopraxia.

Medical Treatment for People with Schizophrenia

Medications and psychotherapy are indicated for patients with schizophrenia. Among the classifications of prescribed medications for certain patients are the antipsychotics and anticholinergic medications. The latter of the two is used to combat the effects of the extrapyramidal side effects of antipsychotics. Psychotherapy includes individual, group, and family therapy.

Electroconvulsive therapy (ECT) is used in some difficult cases; however, it is not used until other methods of therapy have been attempted.

Nursing Interventions for People with Schizophrenia

The goals of nursing interventions include support, structure, consistency, and safety for the patient.

1. Never reinforce hallucinations, delusions, or illusions

It is necessary to keep the patient in reality as *we* know it. Some examples of responses to patients who are hallucinating are listed in Table 13–1.

Table 13–1   SUGGESTIONS FOR HANDLING HALLUCINATIONS IN PATIENTS WITH SCHIZOPHRENIA

SUGGESTED ACTION	RATIONALE
1. "Mr. R, I don't see any snakes. It is time for lunch. I will walk to the dining room with you."	1. Lets the patient know you heard him but immediately brings him into the reality of time of day and the need to go to the dining room.
2. "I see a crack in the wall, Mr. R. It is harmless; you are safe. Susan is here to take you down to occupational therapy now."	2. This is in response to a probable illusion. It lets the patient know that you see something. It validates his fear but tells him what you see and then moves him into the here and now.
3. "I know that your thoughts seem very real to you, Ms. C, but they do not seem logical to me. I would like for you to come to your room and get dressed now, please."	3. Again, you are validating the patient's concern without exploring and focusing on the delusion.
4. "Ms. C, it appears to me that you are listening to someone. Are you hearing voices other than mine?"	4. This is a method of validating your impression of what you see. This is as far as you will go into exploring what she may be hearing.
5. "Thank you, Ms. C. I want to help you focus away from the other voices. I am real; they are not. Please come with me to the reading room."	5. Responds to her in the present and reinforces her response to you. Attempts to redirect her thinking.

2. Never whisper or laugh when patient cannot hear the whole conversation
3. Avoid placing patient in situations of competition or embarrassment
4. Trust
5. Milieu

6.   Communication

KEY CONCEPTS
1.   Schizophrenia is best described as a group of disorders in which people display unusual behavior. There are viable arguments for both psychoanalytic and biologic causes of schizophrenia.
2.   Onset of schizophrenia most often appears in the adolescent or early adult years.
3.   Schizophrenia is a difficult disorder to treat from a medical and a nursing standpoint.

CRITICAL THINKING QUESTIONS
1.   Your 17-year-old nephew who has always been an honor roll student has been earning C and D grades for the last 6 months. He quit the football team, stating that "all the other members were plotting against me." When he sees the results of the high school game on the television sports show, he said, "See, they all know about me." His parents ask you if you think he is taking drugs. What will you say to them? What suggestions will you make? How will you approach your nephew?
2.   You are answering the phone on the midnight shift. A young woman's voice on the other end of the telephone tells you that she has "cut myself just like they told me to. I had to do it; they made me do it. Why won't they leave me alone? What else do they want from me?" What will you say to her? What is your priority? How will you get help to her?
3.   It is a very busy day in the clinic. An adolescent approaches the appointment desk and asks to be seen for a headache. It is possible to work the adolescent in, so you give him or her the patient form to complete and ask him or her to have a seat in the waiting area until called. The television is on. Suddenly, the others begin screaming; you and the staff members arrive at the front desk to see the adolescent wielding a gun and pointing it at the television. He is agitated and says loudly to the television, "You will not control me. I will do what you say and then you will leave me alone. I will shoot if you try again." What will you do first? What will you say? What safety issues must you consider?

SAMPLE QUESTIONS
1.   The main symptom of paranoid schizophrenia is:

   A.   Stupor

   B.   Associative looseness

   C.   Suspicion

   D.   Hyperexcitability

2.   Brian, an 18-year-old who has schizophrenia, is negative, delusional, and withdrawn from others. An appropriate nursing intervention that is appropriate for promoting activity for him is:

   A.   Tell him the voices told you he should participate in the Ping-Pong..fine! game.

   B.   Remind him that he does not want to get worse by sitting alone.

   C.   Tell him he must join the Ping-Pong game; it is part of his care plan.

   D.   Invite him to join the Ping-Pong game.

3. Shawna is a 22-year-old woman who has episodes of extreme muscle rigidity and hyperexcitability. She sometimes repeats a word or phrase over and over. Attempts to move her are met with even more muscle resistance. Shawna probably has what type of schizophrenia?

   A. Catatonic

   B. Disorganized

   C. Paranoid

   D. Schizotypal

4. Mr. Goodbody is calling out, "Nurse!" When you arrive in his room, he tells you to be careful of the snake in the corner. You do not see anything in the corner. Mr. Goodbody is experiencing a(n):

   A. Hallucination

   B. Attention-getting behavior

   C. Illusion

   D. Delusion

5. Of the following responses, which would be your *best* response to Mr. Goodbody regarding the snake?

   A. You say, "Don't worry; I'll get rid of it," as you pretend to remove the snake

   B. "I don't see a snake; what else do you see that isn't there?"

   C. "I don't see a snake. It is time for your group meeting. I'll walk with you to the meeting room."

   D. "Where is it? I hate snakes! Let's get out of here."

6. Which of the following is *not* a sign of a person who has untreated schizophrenia?

   A. Usually experiences a loss of reality

   B. Lives in own world

   C. Functions normally in society

   D. Has delusions and hallucinations

7. A nursing intervention for a person with schizophrenia is:

   A. Reinforce the hallucinations

   B. Keep the person oriented to reality and to the present time

C.   Administer ECT PRN

D.   Encourage competitive activities

8.   Mr. S shouts, "Look at the snakes on the ceiling!" You see some cracks in the plaster. Mr. S is experiencing a(n):

A.   Hallucination

B.   Illusion

C.   Delusion

D.   Flashback

9.   Your best response to Mr. S might be:

A.   "How many snakes do you see, Mr. S?"

B.   "Yes, I see them too. Let's go to the dayroom."

C.   "I see some cracks in the plaster, but not snakes. Let's go to the dayroom."

D.   "I don't think your medication is working. I'll call the doctor."

10.   Ms. Tight is on your unit for treatment of kidney stones. She suddenly walks to the side of the hallway and becomes rigid and immovable. She begins to repeat the same word over and over. You check her medical record and find she has a history of which of the following disorders?

A.   Paranoid schizophrenia

B.   Disorganized schizophrenia

C.   Schizoaffective schizophrenia

D.   Catatonic schizophrenia

ANSWERS AND RATIONALES

1.   Answer: D

Rationale: The main symptom of paranoid schizophrenia is suspiciousness. Options A and D are symptoms of catatonic schizophrenia. Option B is a general symptom of schizophrenia. It is one of Bleuler's "4 A's."

2.   Answer: D

Rationale: Inviting him to the Ping-Pong game brings him into the present and allows him to make the choice for himself. This helps increase self-esteem, as well as diminish other symptoms. Option A reinforces the hallucinations, which is never an appropriate nursing action. B and C are forms of demands, which may cause the patient to revert to negative and possibly aggressive behaviors.

3. Answer: A

Rationale: Shawna's symptoms are consistent with patients who have catatonic schizophrenia. Option D, schizotypal, is a type of personality disorder but not actually a form of schizophrenia.

4. Answer: A

Rationale: This is an example of a hallucination. The patient sees something that is not there, and there is nothing that could be misinterpreted as a snake. That would be an illusion.

5. Answer: C

Rationale: This is the honest response that focuses on returning the patient to reality. The other responses play into the hallucination or border on belittling the patient.

6. Answer: C

Rationale: Patients who have schizophrenia do not function well in society without treatment. Even with treatment, some patients have a difficult time. The "reality" of schizophrenic people is their own reality, and not the norm of society.

7. Answer: B

Rationale: When caring for people who have schizophrenia, it is important to always keep them oriented to reality and the present. It is also important to direct them away from stressful and competitive situations and never reinforce hallucinations. Administering ECT is not a nursing function.

8. Answer: B

Rationale: This time you are dealing with an illusion. There is something on the ceiling and the patient misinterprets what is there.

9. Answer: C

Rationale: Once again, maintaining honesty and reality is the best response.

10. Answer: D

Rationale: These symptoms are characteristic of catatonic schizophrenia.

SUPPORTIVE MATERIALS
1. "Living With Schizophrenia" (videocassette, 1989), Alliance for the Mentally Ill/Minnesota, 970 Raymond Avenue #105, St. Paul, MN 55114.
2. "Surviving in the World of Normals/Living With Someone With Schizophrenia" (2 videocassettes, 1991), Alliance for the Mentally Ill/ Minnesota, 970 Raymond Avenue #105, St. Paul, MN 55114
3. "Understanding and Communicating With A Person Who Is Hallucinating" (videocassette, 1989), Alliance for the Mentally Ill/ Minnesota, 970 Raymond Avenue #105, St. Paul, MN 55114.

REFERENCES

Bleuler, E. (1911). *Dementia Praecox (Emil Kraepelin) or the Group of Schizophrenias* (p. 26). New York: International Universities Press.

Carson, R.C., Butcher, J.N., and Coleman, J.C. (1988). *Abnormal Psychology and Modern Life*, 8th ed. New York: Harper Collins.

Rubin, Z., Peplau, L., and Salovey, P. (1993). *Psychology*. Boston: Houghton Mifflin, pp. 479–480.

LEARNING OBJECTIVES
1.   Define delirium.
2.   Define dementia.
3.   Identify characteristics of delirium.
4.   Identify characteristics of dementia.
5.   Identify medical treatments for patients who have organic mental disorders.
6.   Identify nursing interventions for patients who have organic mental disorders.

KEY TERMS
- Cognitive
- Delirium
- Dementia
- Organic

This chapter discusses two types of cognitive disorders called **delirium** and **dementia**. Delirium and dementia are considered to be **organic**; that is, there is a known or presumed underlying cause.

Delirium and dementia are classified as organic mental syndromes, but Alzheimer's disease, which is primary degenerative dementia, is included in the classification of organic mental disorders. Dementia is a "mental disorder characterized by severe memory loss, disorientation, impaired attention and judgment, and inability to acquire new information" (Rubin, Peplau, and Salovey, 1993). Delirium is an acute condition. It develops quickly, often in response to prescription medications, alcohol, exposure to some toxic environmental substance, fever, or systemic illness.

Etiologic Theories
Psychological theories about potential causes of organic mental disorders include effects of fear, depression, or anxiety. Biologically, dementia can mimic conditions that may be treatable, such as drug toxicity, depression, an electrolyte imbalance, and nutritional complications. Other biologic causes of dementia include aging, severe alterations in temperature (hypothermia or hyperthermia), systemic illness, physical trauma (anoxia), or chemical trauma (carbon monoxide poisoning and drug or alcohol overuse) that affects the brain.

Differential Diagnosis
It should never be assumed that someone is manifesting symptoms of organic mental disorders. Graves' disease (hyperthyroidism), myxedema (hypothyroidism), Huntington's chorea, and diabetes mellitus are some of the metabolic illnesses that may cause patients to show behaviors that would appear to be delirium or dementia. Arteriosclerosis, which is a narrowing of the arteries to the brain, causes a decreased supply of oxygen to the brain. This can lead to a patient's confusion. Systemic infections, nutritional abnormalities, and electrolyte imbalances are also capable of producing dementia-like symptoms in people.

Types
Delirium Due to a Mental Condition
Anesthesia, medications, pain, or just unfamiliar surroundings may be enough to cause this temporary situation.
        Patients who experience delirium may show any of the following symptoms:
- Fogging of consciousness

- Incoherent or slurred speech
- Perceptual disturbances
- Sleep cycle disturbances (this may be related to a person's *normal* routine; be sure that you find out if this is someone—a nurse, perhaps—who normally works nights and sleeps days)
- Either an increase or a decrease in psychomotor activity
- Disorientation
- Memory impairment
- Symptoms that develop within hours or a couple of days and then fluctuate in intensity during the day

Alzheimer's Disease

Alzheimer's is one of a group of dementia disorders called organic brain disorders. It is progressive and irreversible; in other words, it only worsens with time and at this point is incurable.

There are four stages of progression in Alzheimer's disease. Table 14–1 gives some of the signs and symptoms typically associated with each of these stages.

Table 14–1   STAGES AND SYMPTOMS OF ALZHEIMER'S-TYPE DEMENTIA

STAGE	SYMPTOMS
FIRST	• Slight memory loss • May wander and get lost • Disoriented to time and place
SECOND	• Memory loss worsens • Loses ability to make sound judgments or define simple proverbs such as "a stitch in time saves nine." The person will give a very literal translation rather than understand the underlying message of such proverbs. • Neglects personal hygiene, grooming, and health • May show antisocial behavior
THIRD	• "Forgetting" worsens • May not be able to identify own name or recognize family and close friends • May display inappropriate behaviors such as screaming • May start to lose control of bowel and bladder • May become unsteady walking
FOURTH	• Unable to care for self • Unable to walk well, if at all • Incoherent • Totally incontinent • May have seizures

(Adapted with permission from Kalman, N., and Waughfield, C. (1993). *Mental Health Concepts*, ed 3. Albany, NY: Delmar Publishers. (Table 9–7, p. 220.)

Dementia Due to HIV

Realizing that one has acquired an illness from which one cannot recover from can lead to feelings of depression, anger, and frustration. Patients frequently receive antidepressants and other psychoactive medications to help with these feelings. They may require an antiemetic such as prochlorperazine (Compazine), which is also an antipsychotic.

Opportunistic infections (infections that take advantage of an immunocompromised body) are frequent invaders of people who have human immunodeficiency virus/acquired immunodeficiency syndrome (HIV/AIDS). Complications of these infections can cause delirium in people who have HIV/AIDS, just as they can in any other person who gets ill.

As the nervous system becomes involved, people who have AIDS may develop a neuropathy similar to the type seen in patients who have diabetes mellitus. Some relief can be obtained in a person's feeling and functioning with the use of medications such as amitriptyline (Elavil).

Knowledge of the psychotropic medication classifications is very important when working with patients who have AIDS. However, nurses also need to be aware that, as the disease advances, patients will exhibit many of the same symptoms and behaviors as patients with diseases that are organic mental disorders. Among these behaviors are forms of delirium (hallucinations, confusion, forgetting names of people close to them, and so on) and forms of dementia (severely forgetting things, inability to answer questions or process information, and inability to care for personal needs).

Dementia Due to Head Injury
Head injuries cause trauma to the brain that is sometimes reversible and sometimes irreversible. The patient who has sustained a head injury, then, may display signs of either delirium or dementia, or both.

Medical Treatment for People with Organic Mental Disorders
In 1993, the Food and Drug Administration (FDA) approved a medication called THA, or tacrine hydrochloride (Cognex), for treating patients with Alzheimer's-type dementia. Restraints for the patients' safety may be required.

Patients with dementia should be followed closely and treatment regimens change with the patient's condition. Treatment includes diet, medication, and ancillary therapies, such as occupational therapy, physical therapy, and reality orientation.

Nursing Care for People with Organic Mental Disorders
1. Stay calm.
2. Do not argue.
3. Use clear and simple verbal communication.
4. Allow time for patient to respond.
5. Use touch when appropriate.
6. Use restraints when appropriate.
7. Assist with ADLs, as appropriate to the situation.
8. Provide adequate stimulation.

KEY CONCEPTS
1. Organic mental disorders are complex alterations to mental integrity. Dementia and delirium are the two most frequently occurring forms of organic mental disorders.
2. Delirium is usually reversible; dementia is usually irreversible.
3. Nursing care involves safety, honesty, and patience. Medical and nursing interventions are specific to the patient.
4. HIV/AIDS, head injuries, and other medical conditions are not mental health issues. The behaviors of delirium and dementia that may be a result of these medical illnesses require knowledge of mental health principles.

CRITICAL THINKING EXERCISES
1. Uncle J is 65-years-old. He has been picked up by local law enforcement, who found him wandering along the main thoroughfare in your city. He is combative and keeps calling you by his wife's name. Three hours later, Uncle J is reoriented to person, place, and time.

What will you do for Uncle J? Develop a plan of care for Uncle J. What assessments will you make with Uncle J?

2. You are the assistant charge nurse on the Alzheimer's unit. You notice that several patients stop walking when they reach the fire doors on the unit; other residents become visibly agitated when they reach this point in the hallway. You also notice that the carpeting on the other side of the fire doors is a different color. You know that perception changes could be causing some of these reactions. Changing the color of the carpeting is not an option because of cost constraints. How can you help these residents? What nursing actions would be appropriate?

SAMPLE QUESTIONS

1. You are working the night shift in your surgical unit. Ms. Y is one day postoperative for total hip replacement. She is taking several medications for pain and an antibiotic. She is 70-years-old and presented as alert and oriented prior to surgery. She lives independently. Ms. Y suddenly begins screaming and thrashing in bed begging you to "get the spiders out of my bed!" What is the best explanation for Ms. Y's behavior?

   A. Delusions

   B. Delirium

   C. Dementia

   D. Dilemma

2. The best nursing intervention for you, the licensed practical nurse/licensed vocational nurse, to help Ms. Y is:

   A. Inform the charge nurse and doctor immediately.

   B. Turn on the light and ask her where the "spiders" are.

   C. Stop her pain medications.

   D. Check her medical record for a diagnosis of mental illness.

3. Mr. H has been admitted to your nursing home in stage III Alzheimer's disease. Mrs. H is crying and says to you, "Nurse, when will he get better? I don't know what I will do without him home. Why can't the doctor fix him?" Your best response to Mrs. H is:

   A. "Don't worry, Mrs. H. Everything will be fine."

   B. "Relax and enjoy yourself, Mrs. H. You should go out to lunch with your friends and forget about this for a while!"

   C. "Why are you afraid to be home alone, Mrs. H?"

   D. "Mrs. H, your doctor has explained that Mr. H will not get better. How can I help you plan for your future?"

4. Tacrine hydrochloride is a new medication, approved in 1993, for the treatment of symptoms of Alzheimer's-type dementia. Nurses must be alert to results of which of the following side effects?

A. Lowered liver function tests

B. Elevated liver function tests

C. Lowered HDL

D. Elevated TSH

5. Which statement is *not* true about Alzheimer's disease?

A. It is a dementia disorder.

B. It may occur in middle to late life.

C. It is a chronic disease.

D. It is caused by aging and hardening of the arteries.

6. Which of the following would you expect to see in a patient who is diagnosed with an organic mental disorder?

A. Intact memory

B. Appropriate behavior

C. Disorganization of thought

D. Orientation to person, place, and time

7. Ms. P has been admitted to your unit with a diagnosis of a right tibia fracture. Her emergency room notes say that she fell at home. She admits to having "a lot to drink" over the past week. She is disoriented to time, forgets where she is momentarily, is easily distracted, and has a short attention span. She does not answer questions appropriately. She is probably experiencing:

A. Delusions

B. Delirium

C. Dementia

D. Dilemma

8. Your patient who is recovering from an exacerbation of an AIDS-related infection is opting to be treated by family and friends at home. The family has expressed concern because they sense a change in the patient's cognitive abilities. Part of the discharge teaching for this family might include:

A. "It's nothing, really. Patients sometimes get confused in the hospital."

B. "Keep an eye on him or her. You don't want him or her to start wandering."

C. "You're concerned about the change in his or her ability to remember things? Let me call the doctor for you. This is something that you two need to discuss together."

D. "I thought something was strange!"

ANSWERS AND RATIONALES

1. Answer: C

Rationale: Delirium is probably the best choice, as she presented as alert and oriented before surgery. There is no indication at this point that there is dementia. She is not delusional; she is having a hallucination. The dilemma may be what the nurse chooses to do next!

2. Answer: A

Rationale: Your best action is to call your charge nurse/physician immediately. Your state Nurse Practice Act dictates who you should call first. Turning on the light may be helpful but asking about the spiders plays into the hallucination, which is not therapeutic. Stopping her pain medications is not an independent nursing function; you need to make that call to the physician first. Checking her medical record should have been done earlier, but it is not helpful to her right now.

3. Answer: D

Rationale: You have restated what the doctor has already told Mrs. H, you have reinforced reality, and you have been honest. You offered to help her, which shows your concern for her needs. The other choices are all blocks to therapeutic or helping communication.

4. Answer: B

Rationale: Tacrine can elevate liver function tests. TSH is a thyroid-stimulating hormone and HDL is a type of cholesterol.

5. Answer: D

Rationale: Alzheimer's-type dementia is *not* a result of aging or arteriosclerosis. These conditions may be present in addition to the dementia.

6. Answer: C

Rationale: You would expect to see an impaired memory, as well as other impaired cognitive processes in someone who has an organic mental disorder. The person is probably not oriented to at least one of the three spheres of person, place, or time.

7. Answer: B

Rationale: These symptoms are consistent with a person experiencing delirium. The admission of alcohol use adds to this conclusion. Time or decompensation of memory and behavior might change this initial diagnosis to a form of dementia.

8. Answer: C

Rationale: This is the best option. You show concern for the patient, the patient's family, and the situation they are all in. You state the implied message and offer to get the physician, who needs to be the one to give the initial information. You maintain dignity for all and behave professionally.

SUPPORTIVE MATERIALS
1. "Organic Mental Disorders" (videocassette), from the series *The World of Abnormal Psychology*, Annenberg/CPB Collection, P.O. Box 2345, S. Burlington, VT 05407-2345.

REFERENCES

Park, C.C., with Shapiro, L.N. (1976). *You Are Not Alone*. Boston: Little, Brown, and Company, 1976.

Rubin, Z., Peplau, L., and Salovey, P. (1993). *Psychology*. Boston: Houghton Mifflin.

LEARNING OBJECTIVES
1.   Define substance abuse.
2.   Define substance dependence.
3.   Define codependency.
4.   Identify common medical treatments for abuse disorders.
5.   Identify nursing interventions for patients with abuse disorders.

KEY TERMS
- Alcohol abuse
- Alcohol dependence
- Codependent
- Drug abuse
- Drug dependence
- Dysfunctional

Alcoholism and chemical dependency are serious conditions being dealt with in American society.

People start using alcohol and drugs for many reasons, but the main reason is usually to feel accepted by a peer group or to feel comfortable in social situations. Alcohol and other mind-altering chemicals are of high priority because of their prevalence in U.S. society. Approximately $85 billion is spent annually in the United States on alcohol-related conditions (Rubin, Peplau, and Salovey, 1993).

Addiction means physical dependence on a substance. **Substance dependence** is a condition in which a person has had three or more of the following symptoms for 1 month or longer:
- Needs more substance and at more frequent intervals
- Spends a lot of time obtaining the substance
- Gives up important social or professional functions in order to use the substance
- Has tried at least once to quit but still obsesses about the substance
- Misuse or withdrawal symptoms interfere with job, family or social activities
- Uses regardless of the problems created by this use
- Tolerance increases greatly (by approximately 50 percent)
- Uses to avoid withdrawal symptoms

Substance abuse is defined differently than dependence and is diagnosed by a rating system as follows:
- *Mild*-person meets the three of the above symptoms, but social functioning is only minimally affected.
- *Moderate*-person's symptoms are somewhere in between *mild* and *severe*
- *Severe*-more than three of the above symptoms and social obligations are impaired
- *Partial remission*-over 6 months, some symptoms have occurred
- *Full remission*-over 6 months, no symptoms have occurred

Not all patients who abuse substances go through all stages and not everyone will go through them in the same order.

Substance abuse is not a one-person illness; it affects the personal and professional relationships of the people who are associated with the user. A term used to refer to the relationships within an alcoholic family is **dysfunctional**; dishonesty and inability to discuss the situation are strong components. Eventually, this leads to a condition called **codependency**. In codependency, the significant others in the family group begin to lose their own sense of identity and purpose and exist solely for the abuser. Some theorists are using a new term, which includes all kinds of addictive behaviors. They are referring to an "addictive personality" which may begin to explain addictions to food, sex, and gambling as well as alcohol, chemicals and any other dependency that someone develops

Etiologic Theories
Psychoanalytic theories state that people who develop addictions to alcohol or other substances are people who failed to successfully pass through the oral stage of development.

Biologic theories include numerous studies, which imply that there is a familial connection; some sort of metabolic genetic disorder. The cognitive-behavioral theorists suggest that how a person perceives being high may influence the actual act of becoming high.

Differential Diagnosis
Frequently, the alcoholic patient will be admitted to your unit with diagnoses including dehydration, hyperemesis, or respiratory infections.

Types
Alcohol Abuse and Dependence
Alcohol dependence includes improper use of alcohol, impaired social functioning and may show signs of tolerance or withdrawal.

Alcohol abuse usually includes several main symptoms:
1. Pattern of improper use:
   * Daily use/use of more than a fifth of liquor daily
   * Inability to cut down or stop using
   * Binges that last 2 days or more
   * Blackouts (amnesia while intoxicated)
2. Social function is impaired
3. Lasts one month or longer

E.M. Jellinek, who is a pioneer in the area of alcohol use and abuse, has developed another classification for alcoholism. His stages are as follows:
1. Prealcoholic
2. Prodromal
3. Crucial
4. Chronic
5. Other signs and symptoms:
   * Vomiting
   * Dehydration
   * Temper tantrums
   * Disorientation

Treatment Modalities for Alcohol Abuse and Dependency
Treatment for alcohol dependency and abuse is slow. "The single most effective treatment for alcoholism is Alcoholics Anonymous (AA)" (research from the class). There are corresponding groups for families of alcoholics (Al-Anon) and a special group for teenage children (Alateen). Adult Children of Alcoholics is a branch of AA formed for people who are now adults, but who grew up with an alcoholic and were not able to get help at the time.

Rational emotive therapy is being used as well. This type of therapy is based on the belief that it is the way a person perceives being high that makes the difference between use and abuse. Psychoanalysis may also be used, though this is a very costly method of treatment compared to AA, which is free. Family therapy is very important to reinstating the honesty in communication.

Medications are used cautiously. It is not always looked upon wisely to substitute the alcohol with another chemical. Generally, drugs from the antidepressant or antianxiety classifications are prescribed. disulfiram (Antabuse) is a medication that is sometimes prescribed for the person who abuses alcohol.

People who have abused alcohol and are cut off from it suddenly may experience delirium tremens (DTs). In DTs, there is hyperexcitability in the individual's sensory activity. Visual hallucinations (e.g., "pink elephants" and "snakes all over") are common, and tremors and possibly tonic-clonic seizures are typical.

Nursing Care for Treating Patients with Alcohol Dependency and Abuse
1. Honesty
2. Group
3. Awareness of use of defense mechanisms
4. Support
5. Safety
6. Tough love

Drug Abuse and Dependence
Many substances can be addictive to humans. Caffeine and nicotine are two that are very readily available and easy to obtain. It has been said that the single most difficult addiction to overcome is the addiction to nicotine.

It is becoming more and more popular among the youth in the United States to use inhalants such as lighter fluid, paint and paint thinners, and gasoline to get high.

Signs and Symptoms of Drug Abuse and Dependence
- Red, watery eyes
- Runny nose
- Hostility
- Paranoia
- Needle tracks on arms or legs

Treatment Modalities for Patients with Drug Dependence and Abuse
1. Narcotics Anonymous
2. Group therapy
3. Psychotherapy
4. Methadone programs

Nursing Care for Patients with Drug Dependence and Abuse
Nursing care for people who are drug dependent is essentially the same as for those who are alcohol dependent.

KEY CONCEPTS
1. Abuse and dependence on alcohol and other substances is a growing disorder in the United States. Much time and money is being spent on treating the disorders and the illnesses associated with them.
2. Signs and symptoms of alcohol and chemical abuse can be masked as other symptoms. Good observations and careful documentation by the nurse can help to attain the information needed for accurate diagnosis.
3. Medical and nursing care are very similar for both alcohol and drug disorders. It is important to remember that physicians and nurses do not "cure" the person with an addiction. The person must want to be chemically free. Healing must come from within. Physicians and nurses are tools to help the patient learn to do that.

4. Alcoholics Anonymous and Narcotics Anonymous are support groups for people who are chemically dependent. They have a very high success rate, and there are corresponding groups for family members who also need help for the illness.
5. Codependency is also an illness. Codependent people are generally closely linked with the chemically dependent person. People who are codependent need some kind of therapy to help regain their identity and allow the chemically dependent person to again become responsible for his or her own actions.

CRITICAL THINKING EXERCISES
1. Find an "open" AA meeting. Explain that you are a student and ask permission to take notes. Listen and participate if you are invited to do so. Write a short paper on your impressions about the meeting.

SAMPLE QUESTIONS
1. The *desired* effects of disulfiram (Antabuse) include:

    A. Nausea, vomiting, and palpitations

    B. Delirium, impotence, and personality changes

    C. Euphoria, delusions of grandeur, and mania

    D. Hepatitis, gastritis, and esophagitis

2. The defense mechanism most frequently demonstrated by the chemically dependent person is:

    A. Undoing

    B. Rationalization

    C. Denial

    D. Reaction formation

3. The best nursing action for people who are in active withdrawal is:

    A. Tell the patient how destructive the behavior is

    B. Obtain assessment from patient

    C. Explore hallucinations with the patient

    D. Maintain safety for patient

4. Nurses know that alcohol functions as a

    A. Central nervous system (CNS) depressant

    B. CNS stimulant

C. Major tranquilizer

D. Minor tranquilizer

5. The patient who is experiencing delirium tremens (DTs) is most likely to exhibit which of the following types of hallucinations?

A. Auditory

B. Visual

C. Tactile

D. Olfactory

6. Sally and Susie are twins. They are 20-years-old. Susie has a habit of drinking too much when they go out. They were out celebrating their birthdays last night and this morning Susie is vomiting. Sally calls her sister's teacher and says, "Susie is really ill. I think she has the flu; anyway, she can't come to school today. She said she has a test today and an assignment that she was supposed to pick up. I can come in and get the assignment for her. When can she make up the test?" Sally's behavior might indicate:

A. Collaboration

B. Compensation

C. Lying

D. Codependency

7. You are Sally and Susie's friend. A therapeutic response to them might be:

A. "Sally and Susie, you are really going to get in trouble if you keep partying like that. It's bad for you."

B. "Sally and Susie, I care for you both, but Susie, you misuse alcohol. You both need help. Sally, you are not helping Susie by 'taking care' of her; she needs to do it herself."

C. "Sally, why do you keep lying for Susie? Just because she's in trouble doesn't mean you have to cover up for her."

D. "Susie, this is just a stage you're going through. Everybody does it; it's not big deal. You're young! Have fun!"

8. Sally and Susie seek treatment. Susie is treated in-house and Sally is treated as an outpatient. The nurse planning discharge teaching should encourage them to:

A. Attend weekly AA and Al-Anon meetings

B. Check back in to the hospital unit weekly

C.   Attend weekly sessions with the psychologist

D.   Attend weekly Adult Children of Alcoholics meetings

9.   Your patient admits to using an illegal substance daily, thinks about it when not actually using, and spends a lot of time figuring out where to get it. This patient could have:

A.   A delusion

B.   DTs

C.   A dependency

D.   Dementia

10.   One of the major skills a chemically dependent person/family can learn during treatment is:

A.   Honest communication

B.   Codependency

C.   Denial

D.   Scapegoating

ANSWERS AND RATIONALES

1.   Answer: A

Rationale: The desired effects of disulfiram (Antabuse) are supposed to produce nausea, vomiting, and heart palpitations. All other choices are possible side effects.

2.   Answer: C

Rationale: Denial is the most common defense mechanism used by people who are chemically dependent. Rationalization is also seen in some patients.

3.   Answer: D

Rationale: Maintaining safety is very important during DTs or withdrawal. Nurses should never encourage hallucinations. This is not the time for trying to assess the situation or educate the patient. The patient probably does not want to listen, let alone be able to listen, while coming down from the chemical.

4.   Answer: A

Rationale: Alcohol is a CNS depressant. The "high" that people feel is temporary and very misleading.

5.   Answer: B

Rationale: DTs are associated with frequency of visual hallucinations.

6.   Answer: D

Rationale: Sally may very well be codependent in her sister's alcohol abuse. Sally is taking responsibility for Susie's behavior instead of having Susie take care of herself.

7.   Answer: B

Rationale: This response addresses both sisters and tells them that they both need some help. It is honest and caring, and puts the responsibility on them to help themselves through this situation.

8.   Answer: A

Rationale: Susie would be encouraged to attend weekly AA meetings and Sally would be encouraged to attend weekly Al-Anon meetings. We do not know from the information if they *are* adult children of alcoholics; therefore, that would not be the best choice at this time. There is no need to check into the unit weekly, but they can be told that it is acceptable to call or check in if they choose to. The psychologist will tell them the meeting schedule; this would not be a nursing function for discharge planning.

9.   Answer: C

Rationale: The person who is dependent on a substance will display all of these behaviors.

10.   Answer: A

Rationale: Honest communication is necessary in order for the person and family to heal.

ACTIVITY
1.   Most students work, as well as go to school. Have students contact the human resources department where they work or check their employee policy manuals to see what statements are made relating to employing new workers who are chemically dependent *or* what steps are in place to assist current employees who are chemically dependent. Also look into the insurance benefits at the students' employers to determine what coverage is provided for employees who are chemically dependent. Compare and contrast findings as a group discussion.

SUPPORTIVE MATERIALS
1.   "The Meaning of Addiction" (videocassette, 1994), from the series *Thinking Allowed*, 5966 Zinn Drive, Oakland, CA 94611.
2.   "How To Stop The One You Love From Drinking and Using Drugs" (videocassette, 1989), Paramount Pictures Corporation, Hollywood, CA.
3.   "A Gentle Path Through The Twelve Steps" (videocassette, 1989), CompCare Publishers, Minneapolis, MN.

REFERENCES
Rubin, Z., Peplau, L., and Salovey, P. (1993). *Psychology*. Boston: Houghton Mifflin.

LEARNING OBJECTIVES
1.   Define anorexia.
2.   Define bulimia.
3.   Define morbid obesity
4.   Identify populations at risk for eating disorders.
5.   Identify possible causes of eating disorders.
6.   Identify signs and symptoms of eating disorders.
7.   List nursing actions for caring for patients with eating disorders.

KEY TERMS
• Anorexia
• Body image
• Bulimia
• Morbid obesity

Etiologic Theories
The mind-body connection is a strong one that is entwined in all areas of mental health.

Some psychoanalytic theorists would say that at some point in our development, we had negative experiences with our parents or close caregivers. Sigmund Freud would say that anorexic females are afraid of womanhood and heterosexuality; eating is looked upon as an expression of sexual drive (Brumberg, 1988). Females who have developed anorexia seem to have negative feelings toward their mothers. Regression is the defense mechanism that is believed to be activated, resulting in ineffective emotional development.

Biologically, there is the gender difference. Men and women are built differently. Secondly, there are studies pointing toward a genetic link for body build, size, and the amount of body fat.

Another idea posed by biologic theorists is that there is a disturbance in the functioning of the hypothalamus (which regulates eating and sexual activities) or with the neurochemical, dopamine.

In their book *Black Health Library Guide to Obesity*, Mavis Thompson and Kirk Johnson indicate that there may be special concerns about obesity among the African-American population.

Types of Eating Disorders
Anorexia Nervosa
Anorexia nervosa is an aversion to food. Patients refuse to eat.

Symptoms of anorexia nervosa are:
• Excessive weight loss, usually more than 25 percent of body weight prior to the dieting
• Refusal to maintain normal weight
• Intense fear of being fat (consumes only 200 to 400 cal daily)
• Obsessed thoughts
• Excessive exercising
• Shy and introverted personality
• Perfectionism
• Lack of trust in own emotions
• Feeling inadequate and seeing self as fat, no matter what the weight
• Absence of menstrual periods
• Very little sleep (2 or 3 hours per night)

Nursing Interventions for Anorexia Nervosa
1.   Promote positive self-concept
2.   Promote healthy coping skills
3.   Promote adequate nutrition

Bulimia Nervosa
Bulimia is binge eating. People consume huge amounts of food, as much as 8000 cal in a 2-hour period several times daily. A person who is bulimic can consume up to 50,000 cal per day. This is followed by forced vomiting. Bulimia also tends to manifest during adolescence.
   Symptoms of bulimia nervosa are:
- Extreme dieting
- Use and abuse of laxatives or syrup of ipecac (which induces vomiting)
- Use and abuse of diuretics
- Obsessed with food and eating
- Very sensitive to body shape and weight
- Poor self concept
- Thoughts of harming self and possibly suicide
- Impulsive
- Feelings of depression, guilt, and worthlessness
- Erosion of teeth enamel or hoarseness as a result of increased hydrochloric acid from vomiting

Nursing Interventions for Bulimia Nervosa
The nursing interventions for the person who has bulimia are essentially the same as those for the person who has anorexia. In addition, the nurse monitors electrolytes from lab reports and notifies the supervisor and physician for any abnormalities.

Morbid Obesity
Obesity is defined as body weight that is greater than 15 percent of the established ideal height-weight charts. **Morbid obesity**, or hyperobesity, is the condition of being more than 100 lb above ideal body weight. It is associated with the number of fat cells in the body. Biologic reasons for obesity are hypothyroidism and diabetes. Among the negative concepts of obesity is the fact that much of society blames overweight people and assumes that they are weak and lazy individuals.
   The psychoanalytic view of obesity believes that the oral stage of development is the highest level achieved.
   The behaviorists would tell us that food is a mainstay of social and cultural activities; food is a powerful reinforcer.

Complications of Eating Disorders
- Electrolyte imbalances
- Heart irregularities
- Edema and dehydration
- Gastrointestinal problems

KEY CONCEPTS
1.   Eating disorders of one type or another affect large numbers of people in the United States. Statistics primarily reflect women with these disorders; however, men are also becoming more affected with eating disorders as a result of the increase in popularity of male models.

2. Eating disorders are serious and can become fatal as a result of malnutrition and electrolyte disturbances.
3. Eating disorders may have an emotional or physical basis. Obesity per se may have genetic and emotional causes.

CRITICAL THINKING EXERCISES
1. Interview an overweight classmate, family member, or coworker. Ask that person about his or her attempts at weight loss. What was his or her success rate? What was the attitude of the physicians who were helping them? What is his or her perception of the social view of obesity? What is your attitude about people who are overweight? If possible, plan a diet and exercise regimen with the person you interviewed. Be sure that they have the permission of his or her physician before starting the diet and exercise program. Follow and document their progress for this school term.
2. Watch television with a new eye. Which shows are popular? Which commercials appeal to you? What do the characters look like? What roles do thin people play on the shows and commercials? What sells the product on the commercial? How many fat people do you see on these same shows and commercials? What roles do they play? What messages are being sent?

SAMPLE QUESTIONS
1. The eating disorder that is characterized as an aversion to food is called:

   A. Morbid obesity

   B. Bulimia nervosa

   C. Anorexia nervosa

   D. Pica

2. The group of Americans who appear to have the highest percentage of obesity is:

   A. White Americans

   B. Hispanic-Americans

   C. Asian-Americans

   D. African-Americans

3. Your 19-year-old patient has a diagnosis of anorexia nervosa. You notice that he or she seems to spend more time playing with his or her food than eating it. You know that patients with anorexia:

   A. Eat normally if ignored

   B. Fear being fat

   C. Have an accurate body image

   D. Binge and purge

4. An appropriate nursing diagnosis for a patient who has anorexia might be:

   A. Altered nutrition; less than required amount, as evidenced by disinterest in eating

   B. Altered nutrition; more than required amount, as evidenced by eating meals of 2000 cal or more six to seven times per day

   C. Altered body image, as evidenced by stating the wish that others look as good as the patient

   D. Fluid excess related to increased weight gain

5. A key nursing intervention to help patients with eating disorders is:

   A. Let them know that they will be watched closely at meal times

   B. Have patients chart their own intake and output

   C. Insist that patients stay with a staff person for 2 hours after each meal

   D. Encourage patients to express underlying feelings about food, body image, and self-worth

6. Bulimia nervosa is characterized by all of the following *except*:

   A. Bingeing on food

   B. Purging the food after eating it

   C. The ability to control eating pattern

   D. Obsession with body shape and size

ANSWERS AND RATIONALES

1. Answer: C

   Rationale: Anorexia nervosa is the fear of food. Bulimia nervosa is binge eating. Pica is an eating disorder seen in young children.

2. Answer: D

   Rationale: Current statistics point to the African-American group as having a higher percentage of obesity than the national average as a whole.

3. Answer: B

   Rationale: Patients who have anorexia have an intense fear of being fat. They have an inaccurate sense of their size and body image, and will not develop normal eating patterns without much help and behavior modification.

4. Answer: A

Rationale: People who are anorexic will have a nutritional deficit and it is probable that they will also have fluid imbalance, which is caused by the lack of intake and perhaps vomiting. There will also be a body image disturbance, but it is a negative self-perception, not positive.

5.   Answer: D

Rationale: Unlocking the feelings surrounding an eating disorder can be very helpful to the patient and treatment team. Focusing on the food and the destructive behaviors associated with the food puts the emphasis on the wrong place.

6.   Answer: C

Rationale: Patients who have bulimia nervosa cannot control their eating. They binge, purge, and are overly concerned and preoccupied with body shape and size.

ACTIVITY

1.   Many cases of anorexia/bulimia are diagnosed in childhood or adolescence. Work with your school's pediatrics instructor to assign the students to a patient with a diagnosed eating disorder if the opportunity arises. Have students list the challenges they specifically encountered while working with a patient who has an eating disorder.

SUPPORTIVE MATERIALS

1. "Cathy Rigby on Eating Disorders" (videocassette, 1991), Increase Video, Reseda, CA.

REFERENCES

Bailey, D.S., and Bailey, D.R. (1997). *Therapeutic Approaches to the Care of the Mentally Ill*, 4th ed. Philadelphia: F.A. Davis.

Brumberg, J.J. (1988). *Fasting Girls—The Emergence of Anorexia Nervosa as a Modern Disease*. Cambridge: Harvard University Press.

Carson, R.C., Butcher, J.N., and Coleman, J.C. (1988). *Abnormal Psychology and Modern Life*, 8th ed. New York: Harper Collins.

Thompson, M., and Johnson, K.A. (1993). *Black Health Library Guide to Obesity*. New York: Henry Holt and Company.

Chapter 18   SUICIDE

LEARNING OBJECTIVES
1.   Identify main populations at risk for suicide.
2.   Identify myths and truths about suicide.
3.   Identify warning signs of suicide.

KEY TERMS
• Suicide

Suicide is the act of killing oneself purposely (Merriam-Webster, 1994). It is a safe estimate that approximately 39 percent of people over age 65 will attempt suicide. What was once a topic that people preferred to ignore, is now an issue of civil rights. People are demanding the right to choose to end their life when the quality of that life is no longer acceptable.

Risk Groups or Factors
• People who:
  • Have depression
  • Have terminal illnesses
  • Are experiencing loss
  • Are lonely
  • Are unemployed
• Minority groups
• Elderly people, especially elderly white men
• Teenagers (Suicide pacts or "copycat suicides" among some adolescent groups and some religious groups may be a reason for the increase in suicide (Came, 1994).
• Alcohol and chemical abuse
• Religious and cultural influences may affect one's outlook on suicide. A religious group may refuse to bury someone in church or with their full blessing if that person has committed suicide.

The most common methods of suicide are:
• Shooting oneself with guns
• Overdosing with medications or prescription drugs
• Hanging
        Men tend to choose the more violent types of ending their life, whereas women tend to choose the overdose method.

Table 18–1   MYTHS AND TRUTHS ABOUT SUICIDE

MYTHS ABOUT SUICIDE	TRUTHS ABOUT SUICIDE
1. Most people who are suicidal do not leave suicide notes.	1. Approximately 80% do leave a note.
2. Children are not at risk for attempting suicide.	2. Children *do* attempt suicide. They often do not have the means to be successful, however. They will use aspirin or similar substances to attempt an overdose.
3. Once a person has attempted suicide and has been stopped, the person will not attempt suicide again.	3. If someone is convinced that suicide is the only option for them, chances are good that he or she will attempt several times, and may be successful if intervention is not successful.

MYTHS ABOUT SUICIDE	TRUTHS ABOUT SUICIDE
4. Suicide happens when the person is in the depths of depression.	4. It is more likely that the patient will appear happier just before suicide. When someone is deeply depressed, they lack the energy and motivation to end their life.
5. People who slit their wrists or use pills are just asking for attention. They are not really serious about suicide.	5. It is true that these are slower methods of death, however, *all suicide attempts should be taken seriously*. Chances are that these people *are* asking for help and they can be helped if taken seriously at this point.

Some of the signs and symptoms of impending suicide are:
1.   Noticeable improvement in mood
2.   Patient starts giving away personal items
3.   Person starts talking about or becomes preoccupied with learning about death and suicide.
4.   Patients who have difficulty sleeping or who awaken frequently very early in the morning.

Nursing Considerations
The goal is always to prevent the suicide.
1.   *Monitor frequently*. Every 10 to 15 minutes is the usual interval for monitoring suicidal patients.
2.   *Safety*
3.   *Medications*
4   *Communicate*
5.   *Contract*. Develop a "suicide contract" with your patient.
6.   *Crisis intervention*
       Medical and therapeutic management of patients who have attempted suicide depends on the individual and the extenuating circumstances. The person may be on an antidepressant medication. The type of therapy might include individual, group, or family therapy, and possible all three types.

KEY CONCEPTS
1.   Suicide is listed as a leading cause of death among different risk groups in the United States. It crosses cultural, age, gender, and socioeconomic boundaries.
2.   There are many myths surrounding suicide. Nurses need to be aware of the facts and have an understanding of warning signs that may signal suicide.
3.   Safety, communication, and excellent nursing skills may be the tools to prevent a suicide. It is crucial that the nurse is careful with medications when working with people who are at risk for suicide.

CRITICAL THINKING EXERCISES
1.   You are at home alone. The telephone rings. It is your best friend "just calling to say goodbye. I just took a whole bottle of pills and I want to go to sleep. Please talk to me until I go to sleep. You've always been there for me; help me to sleep now." What will you do? What will you say to this friend? Who will you get to intervene? What are your feelings regarding your friend?
2.   A patient in your facility is found unconscious. Heart rate is 50, pulse is 8 and thready, and blood pressure is 90/40. The paramedics transport the patient to the local emergency room where he or she is revived. Results of the workup show large quantities of an

antidepressant medication that is given to several patients on that wing. You remember seeing the patient near the medication cart on several occasions recently. Your supervisor has been doing the medication passes on that wing to help out while the regular staff nurse is on vacation. What actions will you pursue?

3. Your 13-year-old child arrives home from school one day and is obviously upset. His or her best friend has begun "acting weird" in recent weeks and "now only wears black. He or she also listens to weird music and won't talk to us anymore. He or she says we'll soon know what we've done wrong." Your child said several classmates have talked to the principal, but the principal said, "There is really nothing wrong about wearing black and listening to weird music. He or she just needs your friendship now." What are your concerns? What can you do to help your child? What actions can you take as a parent? As a healthcare professional?

SAMPLE QUESTIONS

1. A nursing intervention that is appropriate for a patient who is suicidal is:

    A. Report the patient to the police

    B. Ignore the patient's suicidal comments as "attention getting"

    C. Tell the patient that he or she has "so much to live for!"

    D. Teach healthier problem-solving skills

2. A person is most likely to commit suicide when he or she is:

    A. In deepest depression

    B. Apparently feeling "better"

    C. Confused

    D. Feeling loved and appreciated

3. Your patient tells you, "I am just a burden. Everyone would be better off if I was dead." Nurses should be aware that:

    A. Suicidal talk is just an attention-getting device.

    B. Suicide is an impulsive act; it is not thought out.

    C. Suicidal talk or ideation can lead to suicidal behavior.

    D. Suicidal people seldom really attempt suicide.

4. Mr. P is brought to the hospital by his wife. She states that he has recently been treated for depression but that tonight he is saying, "you and the kids don't need me messing up your lives." Mr. P tells you he has been thinking about suicide for some time now. A nursing diagnosis for Mr. P would be:

    A. Knowledge deficit related to family needs

    B. Ineffective individual coping, as evidenced by manipulation of his wife's feelings

C. Anxiety related to hospitalization

D. Potential for self-directed violence, as evidenced by stating suicidal thoughts

5. Your charge nurse tells you that Mr. P must be placed on suicide precautions. The first intervention you begin is:

A. Placing Mr. P in lockup

B. One-on-one observation at least every 15 minutes

C. Calling the security code over the public address system

D. Allowing Mr. P. to shave and do his bedtime cares

ANSWERS AND RATIONALES

1. Answer: D

Rationale: Teaching skills that help the patient deal with the problems of day-to-day life will be helpful in the long run. Option B is a mistake made by people who believe the myth that some suicide attempts are not serious. Option C is a block to therapeutic communication (disagreeing) and may give false hope. The patient does not see that there is much to live for, or the suicide would probably not have been attempted. Option A is also incorrect because reporting the patient to the police is not required in most communities and could be a threat to the patient.

2. Answer: B

Rationale: People are more likely to carry out the suicide when they appear to feel better. Then, they have the energy to create a plan and carry it out. When they are deeply depressed or confused, they are often not able to think clearly enough to plan and carry out the suicide. When they are feeling loved and appreciated, they are less likely to think about suicide. This may be a temporary feeling on their part, however.

3. Answer: C

Rationale: If a person is talking about suicide, the possibility for carrying it out is very real and must be taken seriously. In very few situations is suicidal ideation a manipulative behavior.

4. Answer: D

Rationale: This man has definite potential for self-harm. He is not attempting to manipulate his wife's feelings, although that may be a result on *her* part.

5. Answer: B

Rationale: Your first action is to place the patient on one-on-one observation. Some facilities accomplish this by having staff members perform rounds at a minimum of every 15 minutes; most facilities assign a staff member to stay with the patient. There is no need to place the patient in lockup at this time, and it is not appropriate to publicize the

114

precautions to the whole facility. It would *not* be appropriate to give him his razor, which would be an implement he could use to perform the suicide.

REFERENCES

Came, B. (1994, October 31). The Last Trip. Three teens die in a shocking suicide. *Macleans'* (Canada), p. 14.

Merriam-Webster Dictionary. (1994). Springfield, MA: Merriam-Webster, Inc.

Shives, L.R. (1994) *Basic Concepts of Psychiatric-Mental Health Nursing*, 3rd ed. Philadelphia: J.B. Lippincott.

LEARNING OBJECTIVES
1.   Discuss concepts of aging.
2.   Define ageism.
3.   Identify five mental challenges for the older adult.
4.   Identify medical treatment for the older adult.
5.   Identify five nursing actions for general care of older patients.

KEY WORDS
- Ageism
- Alzheimer's disease
- Elder abuse
- Elderly
- Geriatrics
- Gerontology
- OBRA

Geriatrics or **gerontology** means the study of older adults. The study of older adults is a specialty area in nursing. The majority of people over age 65 are intellectually intact and are able to care for themselves. Older people are basically mentally healthy; that is, they are able to accept and deal with the changes and losses they are experiencing.

There is a phenomenon called **ageism** occurring in the United States. Ageism is discrimination against a group of people on the basis of their age.

The need for intimacy never leaves us. As human beings, the need to love and be loved is one of the primary needs for survival of the individual and the species. We see elderly people becoming a risk group for **elder abuse** (physical and emotional abuse of older people) inflicted by children or caregivers. The Omnibus Budget Reconciliation Act (**OBRA**) is a federal act that provides standards of care for older adults. One of the provisions of OBRA is ensuring proper assessment of elderly people. It is for this reason that only registered nurses (RNs) conduct or coordinate assessments of elderly people. Other health-care team members help with these assessments by providing input on both the patient's abilities and response to the treatment plan.

Nurses care for the older individual not only in the health-care facility but more and more in the privacy of their own homes. Because of the belief that people will stay healthier and maintain more control of their lives if they are able to stay in their homes, the home health industry is growing.

Alzheimer's Disease and Other Cognitive Alterations
As stated in Chapter 14, this illness most likely gradually takes its toll on the individual for 20 or more years. It is only in the later years that the debilitating effects of the disease become observable.

Cerebrovascular Accident (Stroke)
A cerebrovascular accident (CVA) is a devastating and frightening experience for patients and their families. Some of the mental health issues associated with CVAs are depression and aphasia.

Depression
It is not "normal" to feel depressed all the time when we are older. Major depression in the elderly population can show itself differently than in other age groups. These symptoms are

similar to other afflictions common in the elderly such as drug reactions, electrolyte imbalances, and dementia. Nurses must accurately obtain and document information, and be certain that appropriate medical care is obtained to rule out other ailments.

Medication Concerns

The process of pharmacokinetics is slower and less complete in older people.

Patients who live at home may lose track of their medication routine. They may forget to take medications or forget that they have taken them and take another dose. Nurses also need to be aware of the patient's weight, nutrition, and activity levels. Drug toxicity or overdose can present with symptoms similar to those in other patients who have a mental illness or other physical illness.

Table 19–1 shows some common side effects that drugs have on elderly people, other disorders that may have similar symptoms, and nursing actions that can be performed and then taught to the patient.

Table 19–1   POSSIBLE DRUG SIDE EFFECTS FOR ELDERLY PATIENTS*

SIDE EFFECT	OTHER POSSIBILITIES	NURSING ACTIONS
DRY MOUTH	• Stress response; electrolyte imbalance • Vitamin B deficiency	1. Offer sips of water or ice chips. 2. Offer hard, sugar-free candy (such as lemon drops) if patient is able to suck on them without choking. 3. Oral care with light application of lubricant such as petroleum jelly. 4. Review lab work or call physician.
CONSTIPATION	• Fluid and nutritional deficiency; hemorrhoids or rectal pain • Hypothyroidism	1. Assess diet for fiber and fluid intake. 2. Assess area for signs of hemorrhoids or other inflammation. 3. Assess need for laxatives as ordered by physician. 4. Discuss need for physical activity as condition warrants.
ORTHOSTATIC HYPOTENSION	• Heart disorders	1. Assess vital signs. 2. Teach patient how to get out of bed or chair slowly. 3. Tell patient to stay sitting for a few minutes until dizziness goes away.
URINARY COMPLICATIONS	• Prostate problems • Bladder problems • Uterus problems • Urinary tract infections • Cancers	Tell patient to: 1. Take all medications by 1600 hours. 2. Drink little or no fluids after 1600 hours. 3. Keep track of frequency, amount, color, and odor of urine and abdominal girth.

SIDE EFFECT	OTHER POSSIBILITIES	NURSING ACTIONS
CONFUSION/DISORIENTATION/MENTAL SLUGGISHNESS	• Hypoglycemia • Head injury (from a fall and so on) • Infection/fever • Vitamin deficiency • Transient ischemic attack (TIA) • Brain tumor	1. Give sweetened drink. If still confused after 10 minutes, call physician. 2. Check vital signs for signs of infection. 3. Attempt to validate whether patient has had recent head trauma.
FATIGUE	• Infectious process • Anemia • Hypothyroidism • Stress • Narrowing of coronary arteries	1. Assess vital signs. 2. Assess stress level.
MOOD SWINGS/IRRITABILITY	• Psychological disorders • Electrolyte imbalances	1. Use verbal and nonverbal communication skills to assess cause. 2. Request lab work.

Always report these to your charge nurse, document carefully, and notify the physician if that is allowed for licensed practical nurse/licensed vocational nurse (LPN/LVN) practice in your state.

Paranoid Thinking

This may be a result of fear about the environment.

Insomnia

Insomnia, or inability to sleep, is frequently seen in older adults. It can be a result of many conditions, including depression, fear, pain, urinary incontinence, napping during the day, or sometimes a condition known as "sundowner syndrome," in which the person reverses daytime and nighttime hours.

There are some general skills a nurse learns to use, which will make working with the elderly population more effective.
1. *Respect*
2. *Goal setting*
3. *Patience and understanding*
4. *Humor* (*Caution:* Not everyone appreciates humor and not everyone finds humor in the same things. *Never* embarrass the person.)
5. *Safety*
6. *Independence*

KEY CONCEPTS
1. The concept of old age is changing. People are living longer and better after age 65. Older patients are being cared for in facilities and in their homes. Nurses have an active part in assisting the patient to maintain a good quality of life.
2. Normal conditions of aging include diminished hearing, vision, and other sensory acuity. Alzheimer's disease and other cognitive disorders are not considered a part of normal aging.
3. Afflictions that affect the older adult can be mental, physical, or a combination of these. Medication side effects and drug toxicity can also have the same symptoms, as mental illness that affect elderly people. Accuracy of observation and documentation, and

prompt reporting are crucial to a nurse's responsibility in caring for elderly people. Excellent communication skills are also necessary.

CRITICAL THINKING EXERCISES

1. You are celebrating your retirement when the room goes dark. You wake up in a busy room with lights and noise and many people. You think you recognize some of them and you try to call out to them, but they just stand there and look at you. Someone you don't know is trying to say something to you and keeps shining a flashlight in your eye. Your life partner is crying. What happened to you? Why won't they answer you? What are you feeling now? What do you wish someone would do to help you?

2. Mr. Jacobs is a new resident in your nursing home. He is 76-years-old and has a diagnosis of congestive heart failure (CHF). He has recently fallen at home several times and his adult children are concerned that he will become seriously injured. They have told him that he needs to "go there for a while until you get stronger." They tell the staff members, confidentially, that they plan on this to be a permanent placement and will be selling his home to pay for the care. Mr. Jacobs will be started on digoxin, furosemide, and potassium for the CHF and has an order for acetaminophen with codeine for pain.

    Five days later, Mr. Jacobs has had a mood change. His family comes to visit and finds that he is combative and forgetful. One of his children is crying and looks at you and says, "What have you done to him? He's never been like this before." What thoughts cross your mind? How do you respond to this personal attack? How will you attempt to resolve this situation? How would you like to be treated if you were the family member?

SAMPLE QUESTIONS

1. One effective communication technique for assisting a patient with aphasia is:

    A. Try to guess the word or finish the sentence

    B. Associate the word with the object

    C. Tell the patient to think about it while you make the bed

    D. None of the above

2. According to OBRA, who is responsible for completing the assessment of an older adult?

    A. All health staff members

    B. Nursing assistants

    C. LPN/LVN

    D. RN

3. Mrs. Brown, who is usually alert and oriented, is showing signs of confusion. Her vital signs are all within normal limits. She has recently been started on furosemide for CHF. The nurse suspects:

    A. Just normal aging

    B. Stroke

C. A medication side effect

D. Depression

4. A 73-year-old patient in your long-term care center has become withdrawn and cranky. You try to find a method to initiate communication and activity with the patient. Which of the following statements would be the best choice to try communicating with your patient?

A. "Why are you staying over here by yourself?"

B. "Your daughter wants you to make friends here."

C. "I need a partner for the card game; I'd like to have you be my partner."

D. "The doctor said the more you do, the better off you'll be."

5. "Losses" that are associated with the process of aging frequently cause:

A. Presbycusis

B. Depression

C. Dementia

D. CHF

6. When an older patient begins to show signs of dementia, physicians and nurses should assess all of the following *except*:

A. Medication routines

B. Nutritional intake

C. Circulatory function

D. Behaviors that are assumed to be part of normal aging

7. The speech impairment that affects people who have had a stroke is called:

A. Affect

B. Aphasia

C. Autism

D. Ageism

8. Nurses understand that one of the reasons why older people become toxic from their prescription medications is:

A. Drugs are metabolized faster in older people.

B. Drugs are metabolized more slowly in older people.

C. Drugs are ineffective in older people.

D. Drugs need to be ordered in stronger doses for older people.

9. Your patient is admitted with bruises on this head and upper arms. His son is with him and jokes about the bruises, stating, "Dad is getting so clumsy. He falls out of his wheelchair a lot." You glance at the patient, who says nothing, is looking down, and is avoiding eye contact. You become alert for the possibility of:

A. Blood dyscrasias

B. Vitamin deficiency

C. Elder abuse

D. Self-inflicted wounds

10. The federal law that mandates special care and assessment skills for the older population is called:

A. OBE

B. OPRAH

C. COBRA

D. OBRA

ANSWERS AND RATIONALES

1. Answer: B

   Rationale: Reinforce the word by showing or handling the object. Trying to guess the word or finishing the patient's sentence can frustrate and insult the patient, as well as discourage he or she from attempting to stimulate communication. Asking the patient to think about what they want to say it while you do something else is distracting.

2. Answer: D

   Rationale: The federal regulations of OBRA require that the assessment be conducted by a registered nurse for purposes of consistency. All other people on the health-care team supply input and documentation that assist with the assessment.

3. Answer: C

   Rationale: A medication side effect would be the most obvious possibility since the medication is a recent change in the patient's routine and normal vital signs should rule out the possibility of a recent stroke. Depression is a distant possibility.

4. Answer: C

Rationale: You are assertive and tell the patient what you want, in a way that encourages the patient to participate in a specific activity. This statement also supports the person's self-esteem.

5.   Answer: B

Rationale: The losses that people experience as they age are frequent causes of depression.

6.   Answer: D

Rationale: Dementia is *not* a part of normal aging. Other possibilities for unusual behavior should be ruled out before giving someone a diagnosis of dementia.

7.   Answer: B

Rationale: Aphasia is the speech complication that often results from a stroke. Affect can also change after a stroke, but it is not a speech difficulty.

8.   Answer: B

Rationale: Drugs are metabolized more slowly in older people. This results in a cumulative effect that leads to toxicity.

9.   Answer: C

Rationale: These could be symptoms of elder abuse. The location of the bruises is consistent with being shaken or beaten. The lack of eye contact and no verbal response is consistent with the elderly person's fear that the beating might get worse.

10.   Answer: D

Rationale: OBRA is the law that attempts to provide consistency in assessment and care of the aging.

ACTIVITY

1.   While on a medical-surgical or geriatric clinical rotation, have students copy all medications for a patient who is 60-years-old or older. Graph out the "usual adult dose" for each of that patient's medications. Using the 25 percent rule (older adults should, in general, take 25 percent of the usual adult dose), calculate what the patient should be taking. What are your findings? How many patients are receiving the appropriate dose for an older adult? How many patients would you need to call the physician about? What are some rationales for using a higher (or the usual) adult dose of a medication for a particular patient?

REFERENCES
Barry, P.D. (1994). *Mental Health and Mental Illness*, 5th ed. Philadelphia: JB Lippincott.

LEARNING OBJECTIVES
1.   Define homelessness.
2.   Identify some possible reasons for homelessness.

KEY TERMS
- Homeless

Some people are **homeless** as a result of the health-care delivery system. Mentally ill people comprise approximately 50 percent of the homeless in the United States. Many of these people have schizophrenia. Because of the diagnostic criteria, the availability of benefits for the mentally ill, and the nature of the various illnesses, people with certain illnesses have a difficult time living independently with their illness. They end up out of work, out of money, and out of a home.

A small number of people choose to live on the streets. They are making a statement about the priorities of a nation that they think is not serving its people as it said it would. The largest group of people who use community-based mental health services are the poor, especially the homeless poor. (Barry, 1994).

In the 1950s, deinstitutionalization led to the discharging of people who were technically able to be "in the community" but who were not always able to cope with the stresses of caring for themselves and their families, and maintaining employment. For some mentally ill people, this kind of pressure and competition are the factors that keep them ill.

As of 1984, the Department of Housing and Urban Development (HUD) statistics counted approximately 350,000 homeless people in the United States.

In 1987, the Health Resources and Services Administration—Health Care for the Homeless (HRSA-HCH) was formed to provide information and help create plans to help those who were homeless. The problem was, funding of federal programs depends on numbers, and it is extremely difficult to get accurate numbers because they change markedly approximately every two months (*Society Magazine*, 1994).

Most experts, however, believe that 25 to 50 percent of adult homeless people have a psychosis and that 33 to 50 percent are alcoholics (Keltner, Schwecke, and Bostrom, 1991). Schizophrenia is also a major problem among the homeless population. Patients may be brought into your facility through the emergency room or by the law enforcement agencies. Sometimes medication is given to stabilize people, and they are returned back to the communities; sometimes the people are admitted to medical units.

What techniques do you need to help patients who may be homeless and physically or mentally compromised?
1.   Treat the whole person, not the homelessness.
2.   Treat the person as any other person on the unit.
3.   Maintain all patient rights.

CRITICAL THINKING EXERCISES
1.   Review your facility's policies on caring for the homeless. You are the administrator of your facility and you are also a nurse. You are responsible to the board of directors, as well as for the welfare of your patients. What suggestions can you make to improve the treatment that homeless patients receive? How will you adjust your budget, (which is already stretched to the limit), to accommodate your building, patients, staff members, and the special needs of a growing population of chronically ill homeless people?

2. You are the only source of income for your family. You are laid off from your position due to a merger of two agencies. How long can you survive with no income? How will you pay for insurance? Jobs are not plentiful; the outlook for comparable employment in the near future is bleak. How close are you to living on the street? What is your plan of action for you and your family?

SAMPLE QUESTIONS

1. Homelessness is blamed, in part, on:

    A. Deinstitutionalization

    B. Access to community services

    C. Mental illness

    D. All of the above

2. One reason a homeless person might be denied care at a shelter for homeless people is:

    A. He or she has been there too frequently.

    B. He or she is under the influence of alcohol or drugs.

    C. He or she has symptoms of a communicable disease.

    D. All of the above.

ANSWERS AND RATIONALES

1. Answer: D

    Rationale: Deinstitutionalization was intended to be helpful to patients and taxpayers, but it left some people without access to services. Fifty percent of the people who use community-based mental health services are the homeless poor, but other services are hard to access. Having a mental illness makes it difficult for many homeless people to hold jobs that pay enough to support themselves in the community, even with the benefit of having public housing.

2. Answer: B

    Rationale: Most shelters are equipped to take care of ill people either on-site or at a different cooperating agency. Frequency is not usually an issue because shelters work on a first-come–first-served basis. Shelters usually prohibit residency of someone who is under the influence of drugs or alcohol. They are often refused care in the shelter, but offered to be taken to detoxification. When they are no longer under the influence of these substances, they are welcome at the shelter.

ACTIVITY

1. Participate in the evening-out sleepouts, which many major communities participate in as a fundraiser for shelters and food shelves.

SUPPORTIVE MATERIALS
Videos
1. "Dr. Paul Carling on Housing" (videocassette, 1989), Alliance for the Mentally Ill/Minnesota, 970 Raymond Avenue #105, St. Paul, MN 55114.
2. "A Place Called Home" (videocassette, 1990), PBS Productions/Virginia Wolf Productions, Washington, DC.
3. "Down and Out In America" (videocassette, 1987), Joseph Feury Productions/MPI Home video, Oak Forest, IL.

REFERENCES
Barry, P.D. (1994). *Mental Health and Mental Illness*, 5th ed. Philadelphia: J.B. Lippincott.

Keltner, N.L., Schwecke, L.H., and Bostrom, C.E. (1991). *Psychiatric Nursing: A Psychotherapeutic Management Approach*. St. Louis: Mosby-Year Book.

Rossi, P.H. (1989). Down and Out in America—the Origins of Homelessness. Chicago: University of Chicago Press.

Society Magazine (1994, November/December). Social science and the citizen: Counting homelessness. *32*, 2.

Stephens, D., Dennis, E., Toomer, M., and Holloway, J. (1991). The Diversity of Case Management Needs for the Care of Homeless Persons. In Goodnight, G.T. (Ed.), *Homelessness: A Social Dilemma—A Critical Analysis on the Question of Homelessness in the United States*. Chicago: National Textbook Group.

LEARNING OBJECTIVES
1.   Define abuse.
2.   Define victim.
3.   Differentiate between different kinds of abuse.
4.   Identify characteristics of an abuser.
5.   Identify nursing actions to help survivors of abuse.

KEY TERMS
- Abuse
- Abuser
- Date rape
- Elder abuse
- Emotional abuse
- Incest
- Neglect
- Physical abuse
- Rape
- Respite care
- Safe house
- Sexual abuse
- Sexual harassment
- Spouse abuse
- Survivor
- Verbal abuse
- Victim

Abuse is defined by Merriam-Webster (1994) as "1. a corrupt practice, 2. misuse (drug), 3. coarse and insulting speech, 4. mistreatment (child)" and as "1. to put to a wrong use: misuse, 2. mistreat, 3. to attack in words, 4. revile."
        Victim is defined by Webster as, "1. a living being offered as a sacrifice in a religious rite, 2. an individual injured or killed (as by disease or accident), 3. a person cheated, fooled or injured." The experts who work in the field of abuse are divided regarding the term "victim." It connotes a dependency that many believe serves to place the target of abuse in a more dependent position emotionally. Many prefer to use the term **survivor**. It is more positive and forward-thinking than the somewhat defeatist "victim." Both terms are used interchangeably in this text.
        There are strong cultural influences surrounding abuse issues. One of the reasons that abuse is so hard to prosecute is because it is so individualized. People are generally abused by someone close to them, such as a parent, relative, child, spouse, baby-sitter, member of the clergy or some other trusted person.
        Abuse covers all ages, races, walks of life, and economic classes. It does not discriminate according to gender. Statistics are skewed somewhat in favor of female abuse, primarily because men have been reluctant to report abuse by women.

Characteristics of Abusers
1.   Abused himself/herself
2.   Low self-esteem/need for power
3.   Alcoholic/chemically dependent people
4.   Parents of unwanted children

Characteristics of the Victim
1. Dependent or codependent personality
2. Reliant on abuser

Categories of Abuse
1. **Sexual abuse**
    - **Sexual harassment**
    - **Incest**
    - **Rape**
    - **Date rape**
2. **Physical abuse**
3. **Emotional abuse**
4. Child abuse/neglect
    Abuse is an act of *commission*, meaning an act of *doing*. **Neglect** in child abuse or elder abuse is an act of *omission*, or *not doing* something that should be done.
5. **Spouse abuse**
    There are three stages of the abuse cycle that are very prevalent in spouse abuse. They are:
    1. Tension
    2. Serious beating
    3. Honeymoon (Walker, 1979)
6. **Elder abuse**

Nurses and social workers also serve as resource people for families or other caregivers who are caring for the elderly.
Respite care (*Note to teacher:* I have left this area blank, so that you can customize your own discussion of this topic.)

General Criteria for Suspecting Abuse
1. Bruising
2. Bleeding
3. Absence from work or school
4. Depression
5. Withdrawal from friends and social activities
6. Frequent bladder infections
7. Physical abnormalities
8. Frequent visits to the emergency room

General Nursing Actions to Help Abused Persons
1. Ensure safety
2. Know your own thoughts and feelings about abuse
3. Remain nonjudgmental/show empathy
4. Know your agency policy

CRITICAL THINKING EXERCISES
1. Contact an emergency room or clinic in your town. Request an appointment to interview the staff members regarding their policies and procedures for treating abused persons.
2. You go to your neighbor's house for a family party. You notice their 3-year-old son off by himself. You know he is usually eager to play with other children, but this evening he seems particularly shy of your 7-year-old son. An hour later, you notice they are both

gone. You find your son "playing doctor" with the neighbor's 3-year-old. What do you do?

3. Mrs. Jones leaves your long-term care facility for a weekend with her daughter and son-in-law. She seems apprehensive but tells you she is "just worried that I'm a bother to them." You bathed her and helped her pack, and now you document that she has gone until Sunday afternoon and that you were concerned about her apprehension. You noted no other physical or mental abnormalities. Sunday afternoon, she returns with skin tears on both arms and a bruise over her right eye and on her right cheek. She is crying. Her daughter says, "Doesn't that look awful? Gram took a tumble from the toilet." "Gram" says nothing until her daughter leaves, then says to you, "I worry about her. Her husband is a nice man, but he gets so mad at us sometimes. I really can't blame him; he has a lot on his mind, and I can't give them any more money." What are your responsibilities according to your facility? According to your state? According to you personal belief system?

4. You are the licensed practical nurse/licensed vocational nurse working with the registered nurse (RN) on a plan of care for the two patients listed in the previous exercises. List one short-term goal and five nursing interventions that you can suggest to the RN for *each* patient.

REVIEW QUESTIONS

1. When caring for someone who has been abused, the nurse can be therapeutic by:

   A. Showing empathy

   B. Ensuring safety

   C. Contacting counselors and advocates

   D. All of the above

2. Which of the following is a legal requirement for you (the nurse) to perform when caring for a rape victim?

   A. Ask the patient why it happened

   B. Document the information in the patient's own words

   C. Offer to take the patient home after your shift

   D. None of the above

3. When a survivor of abuse and the abuser both present at your facility, your responsibility is to care for:

   A. The survivor only

   B. The abuser only

   C. Both people

   D. Neither one; call the physician

4. A young mother comes to your clinic with her 2-year-old daughter. The mother is crying and distraught. She explains that she is divorced from the child's father, but he has visitation rights. Tonight, when the little girl came back from her father's house, the mother noticed blood on the little girl's panties. She wants to know what to do. Your first action is to:

   A. Get them a good lawyer

   B. Show empathy and offer privacy

   C. Call the police

   D. Tell them you understand just how they feel

5. The little girl is not talking to you or the social workers. You suggest giving her some toys and drawing materials. Your rationale for this is:

   A. It gives you one less person to work with at the moment.

   B. You know children can be bribed.

   C. You think she might talk if she was distracted.

   D. Children often communicate their feelings through play.

6. Mrs. X has been caring for her mother at home. Mrs. X's mother has stage III Alzheimer's disease and requires more of Mrs. X's time. Mrs. X says to you, "I just don't know what to do. I can't stand it anymore. I love my mother, but I don't have any time for myself and I can't afford a nursing home." You say:

   A. "Mrs. X, hang in there. Things have a way of working out."

   B. "Why don't your sisters and brothers help out a little?"

   C. "There are agencies that provide respite care for people in your situation. If you like, I could tell the social worker that you would like some information on this service."

   D. "It's got to be hard to put up with this all day when you aren't trained for it."

ANSWERS AND RATIONALES

1. Answer: D

   Rationale: Showing empathy, offering to provide further assistance, and reassuring safety helps the patient to trust you and probably be more comfortable and compliant with the examinations.

2. Answer: B

   Rationale: Getting a statement in the patient's own words and documenting it in the medical record is required. Option A is information that the patient may not know. The word "why" is counterproductive in therapeutic communication. Option C is not recommended for reasons of liability for both the nurse and the patient. Offering to take

129

the patient home is most likely a violation of your agency policy, as well as a violation of professional ethics.

3.   Answer: C

Rationale: You need to be helpful to both people. You need to take care of the physical and emotional health of both patients, and care for the patients according to the degree of immediacy. A physician needs to be called if there is not one in the immediate area, but until the physician is there, your nursing care, observations, and documentation helps to ensure the best possible care for the patients.

4.   Answer: B

Rationale: Offering empathy and providing privacy helps to calm the mother. Options A and C might be done later, but at the mother's discretion. Option D is not an appropriate choice because it is a block to therapeutic communication. The nurse does not know "just how they feel." This statement is belittling.

5.   Answer: D

Rationale: Children often act out or draw what is troubling them. Offering them toys or drawing materials, and discreetly observing them can tell you much about what they have experienced. These activities may also serve as a diversion, but the purpose of offering toys is to encourage children to express themselves, not to divert attention from the situation.

6.   Answer: C

Rationale: You let Mrs. X know that you have heard her concerns and her need for help. You offer the best help you can at the moment, yet you allow her to make the decision about speaking to the social worker.

ACTIVITY
1.   Choose either Critical Thinking Exercise 1 or 2 from this chapter and have your students write a teaching plan. You can decide which of the people in the scenarios the students should write plans for, since everyone in them can use some guidance.
2.   Invite a representative/advocate from your local abuse prevention or crisis center to speak during a class period. Find out what services are provided, what role the law enforcement and courts play, what a restraining orders do and how they are obtained, and so on. Advocates usually have access to short videos depicting abuse. Request that they bring a video to show the students. (Warning: these can be graphic.) Chances are that at least one person in your class has been abused. Permit the students to feel free to leave for a few moments if they become overwhelmed. If students leave, be prepared to check on them immediately and provide support.

SUPPORTIVE MATERIALS
1.   "Child Abuse: The Perfect Crime" (videocassette, 1989), Houston Public Television, Alexandria, PA.
2.   "Healing Sexual Abuse: The Recovery Process" (videocassette, 1991), Community Television of Southern California/KCET Video.

REFERENCES

Bass, E., and Davis, L. (1993). *Beginning To Heal—The First Book for Survivors of Child Sexual Abuse*. New York: Harper Perennial/Harper Collins.

House Select Committee on Aging. (1991). *Congressional Quarterly Almanac*, 102nd Congress, 1st Session, Washington, DC: CQ Inc.

Keltner, N.L., Schwecke, L.H., and Bostrom, C.E. (1991). *Psychiatric Nursing: A Psychotherapeutic Management Approach*. St. Louis: Mosby-Year Book.

Lachs, M.S., and Pillemer, K. (1995, February 16). Current concepts—Abuse and neglect of elderly persons. *N Engl J Med, 332*: 437–443.

Merriam-Webster. (1994). *The Merriam-Webster New Edition Dictionary*. Springfield, MA: Merriam-Webster.

Rubin, Z., Peplau, L., and Salovey, P. (1993). *Psychology*. Boston: Houghton Mifflin.
Walker, L. (1979). *The Battered Woman*. New York: Harper and Row.

Testbank Questions

Basics of Communication

1. Mr. R., age 60, is admitted to the medical floor for chest pain, which has been diagnosed as probable myocardial infarction (MI). As you are taking him to the room, he states, "I don't know why you're all making such a fuss. This happens all the time. Nothing is wrong. It's just something I ate." The defense mechanism he exhibits is
A. Denial
B. Dissociation
C. Compensation
D. Transference
ANS: A
Response: The patient is denying the situation and the facts as they are happening.
Chapter: Basics of Communication

2. The nurse can most effectively communicate with Mr. R by
A. Stating personal experiences relating to chest pain
B. Finishing his sentences when he hesitates in his speech
C. Maintaining eye contact with him while he speaks
D. Telling him not to worry because that will increase his discomfort
ANS: C
Response: Eye contact is an effective method for showing interest and concern. The nurse can also observe nonverbal communication through eye contact; however, consider the culture of the patient and nurse. Eye contact is a sign of disrespect in some cultures. In this situation, the nurse must ask the patient about the lack of direct eye contact.
Chapter: Basics of Communication

3. In an effort to be helpful, you tell a patient that "everything will be just fine; you'll see." You have broken therapeutic communication by:
A. Agreeing
B. Reassuring the patient with a cliché
C. Disapproving
D. Changing the subject
ANS: B
Response: You have given in to the social response. In therapeutic conversation an overused statement gives the patient a false sense of hope.
Chapter: Basics of Communication

4. When preparing a care plan for a patient with aphasia, which of the following is the best nursing intervention?
A. Immediately correct all mispronounced words
B. Assume that the patient cannot communicate
C. Associate words with objects
D. Speak for the patient if he or she takes too long to answer
ANS: C
Response: Associating words with objects reinforces the patient's learning and ability to make the correct choice. This association also helps the patient to maintain independence in communication.
Chapter: Basics of Communication

5. Mrs. L. has been admitted for a medical work-up to rule out breast cancer. She has been refusing to answer questions while you attempt an assessment. She suddenly states, "You are all so incompetent. How did you ever get a nursing license?" You are aware that she is experiencing some emotional turmoil and you say (therapeutically):
A. "This is very inappropriate behavior, Mrs. L."
B. "I'd like to help, Mrs. L. Please tell me the reason for your anger."
C. "Everyone here is highly educated and qualified, Mrs. L."
D. "Mrs. L., statements such as that are not tolerated here."
ANS: B
Response: This choice combines an assertive statement of the nurse's desire to be helpful and the nurse's statement of an implied or obvious emotion/behavior from the patient.

6. K.C. says that she is so depressed and she does not want to live if she has to wear a colostomy bag for the rest of her life. K.C. says, "I'd just like to end it all." You respond:
A. "Lots of women have colostomies, K.C. It's not so bad."
B. "I know just how you feel, K.C."
C. "You really shouldn't dwell on it, K.C."
D. "End it all? Are you thinking of killing yourself, K.C.?"
ANS: D
Response: The nurse has "parroted" the patient's words of "end it all" and very bluntly uses a closed-ended question to assess the patient for suicidal ideation. In this case, the closed-ended question is acceptable because it follows the patient's specific statement, which the nurse chooses to pursue.
Chapter: Basics of Communication

7. When a period of silence occurs in a therapeutic interaction, the nurse
A. Leaves the room because the conversation is over
B. Quickly changes the subject to talk about as many subjects as possible
C. Sits quietly for a short time to allow both himself or herself and the patient to collect their thoughts
D. Informs the patient that he or she is busy and to put on the call light when the patient is ready to answer more questions
ANS: C
Response: Silence is a beneficial technique that allows both nurse and patient time to collect their thoughts and see what direction the conversation will take.
Chapter: Basics of Communication

8. A young adult patient attempts to manipulate you and other staff. The nurses perceive that this patient is attempting to have his or her needs met. In an attempt to therapeutically interact with the patient, you say:
A. "It is not appropriate for me to do what you want now, but I'd like to stay and talk about it."
B. "This manipulation must stop."
C. "If you attempt to manipulate me again, I will put you in the locked unit."
D. "We all know what you are trying to do."
ANS: A
Response: This honest and assertive statement tells the patient that the nurse is maintaining the therapeutic boundary or the boundary set up by the care plan. The statement also clearly states that the nurse is there to be helpful in other ways.
Chapter: Basics of Communication

9. A patient who has been on your station for several weeks is experiencing rapid advancement of his or her cancer and death is imminent. Which of the following interventions is of highest priority?
A. Monitor vital signs and be alert for changes in physical condition
B. Encourage the patient to talk about his or her feelings regarding death
C. Encourage family members to leave for awhile, so that they and their loved one can rest
D. Contact the attorney (per the family's request) to tie up personal business
ANS: A
Response: Even though it is very important to attend to the patient's mental and emotional peace, the priority of the nurse must always be the patient's physical condition and the documentation of all information and changes in the patient's status.
Chapter: Basics of Communication

10. Patient X. is unhappy about being hospitalized and makes no attempt to conceal that fact by blaming the staff and labeling all of the nurses "stupid" and "incompetent." Patient X. does not cooperate with the plan of care. Your best therapeutic nursing response to patient X. is:
A. "Patient X., this kind of nurse-bashing is very inappropriate."
B. "Patient X., I have some time and I'd like to talk to you about what is angering you."

C. "Patient X., if this continues I will ask to have you confined in the locked unit until you cooperate."
D. "Patient X., all of the nurses here are highly trained professionals."
ANS: B
Response: Offering yourself to listen and help is the most therapeutic choice.
Chapter: Basics of Communication

11. Lilly is in the end stage of cancer. She has been on your medical unit several times and you have developed a trusting relationship with her. Lilly has lost interest in daily activities and seems depressed. She says to you, "What's the use? I'm going to die soon. There's no point in all of this anymore." The most therapeutic response to Lilly is:
A. "Oh, Lilly, don't say that. Worrying doesn't help!"
B. "Lilly, we all feel hopeless sometimes and they're finding new cures all of the time!"
C. "You sound as though you've given up all hope, Lilly. I am concerned about you."
D. "Are you afraid to die, Lilly?"
ANS: C
Response: This response shares your sense about the feelings and thoughts implied by the patient, and shares your empathy; however, it remains open-ended. Option "D" poses a direct question about her feelings but it may be premature, because she has not expressed "fear" in her statement. It is also a closed-ended format.
Chapter: Basics of Communication

12. You are working in pediatrics and are admitting a 4-day-old infant who has spiked a fever of unknown etiology. The child is the first born of a 16-year old single mother. The mother says, "This is a punishment. I feel so guilty for making my baby sick." Your best therapeutic response to her is:
A. "Why do you think you are being punished?"
B. "This is not about you right now. Your baby is sick and needs you!"
C. "It's normal for new mothers to feel guilty. You'll learn not to let it bother you so much!"
D. "I understand your feelings, but this is a physical condition which you did not cause. It is not a punishment!"
ANS: D
Response: This shows the nurse's empathy while reassuring the mother that she is not being punished for anything, as the mother had stated.
Chapter: Basics of Communication

13. A patient has lost the capacity to verbalize his or her needs. As the nurse caring for this patient, you
A. Encourage the patient to use words and to point to objects
B. Continue to use technical terminology in an effort not to "talk down" to the patient
C. Talk to the family and have them answer for the patient
D. Encourage the patient to speak only during speech therapy, in an effort to maintain consistency for the patient
ANS: A
Response: It is important to have the patient maintain as much independent communication as possible. Allowing time for the patient to repeat words, thinking of the correct words, or pointing to the object as you reinforce the word are important techniques to use.
Chapter: Basics of Communication

14. You are caring for a patient with laryngeal cancer who is scheduled for a total laryngectomy in the morning. In your preoperative teaching with the patient and family, your primary focus is:
A. Methods to control pain
B. Methods of payment for extended hospital stay
C. Alternative communication methods
D. Length of the surgery
ANS: C
Response: The patient is potentially concerned about all of the options, but it is of primary concern to make the patient aware of the changes, which will need to be made in communication. It is important to agree upon some "codes" that can be used to communicate initially after surgery. This can also be done with a speech therapist.
Chapter: Basics of Communication

15. Which of the following blocks to therapeutic communication is a nurse displaying when he or she says, "Don't worry about a thing. Everything will turn out for the best"?
A. Disagreeing
B. Belittling
C. Agreeing
D. Reassuring cliché
ANS: D
Response: This is offering false hope by using a phrase repeated frequently in social communication, which has little or no meaning therapeutically.
Chapter: Basics of Communication

16. You are caring for a patient who has had a stroke. Your patient has difficulty communicating verbally or in writing. This type of challenge to the patient's communication is called:
A. Global aphasia
B. Dysphagia
C. Expressive aphasia
D. Receptive aphasia
ANS: C
Response: *Expressive aphasia* is difficulty expressing oneself either verbally or in writing. *Receptive aphasia* is the type of aphasia that interferes with a person's ability to interpret or understand verbal/written communication. *Global aphasia* is a combination of expressive and receptive. *Dysphagia* refers to one's ability to swallow.
Chapter: Basics of Communication

17. Ms. M. is deaf. She is new to your transitional care unit (TCU). Staff has tried to use sign language in an attempt to communicate with her. Ms. M.'s response is to become agitated and walk away. Alternative attempts to communicate with her might include:
A. Offer her a pen and pad of paper
B. Face Ms. M directly and speak normally
C. Use pictures
D. All of the above
ANS: D
Response: All of the above. Not all people who are deaf can use sign language and many can read lips, but exaggerating the words may distort the word and the person may not understand. Offering pictures, especially in the case of difficult ideas that need to be communicated or in the situation of a person with other communication barriers may offer another solution.
Chapter: Basics of Communication

Ethics and Law

1. The licensed vocational nurse/licensed practical nurse (LPN/LVN) knows that his or her scope of practice includes all of the following *except*:
A. Administering nursing care under the direction of a registered nurse (RN)
B. Documenting the patient's data
C. Independently ordering medications for the patient
D. Assisting the physician or registered nurse with more complex care and procedures
ANS: C
Response: Neither RNs nor LPN/LVNs are allowed to "independently" order medications. This is a medical function, not a nursing function. Nurse practitioners may prescribe medication in some states, but they do so under a specific physician's protocol.
Chapter: Ethics and Law

2. The patient is semiconscious and is in need of emergency surgery to relieve a subdural hematoma. The nurse knows that:
A. Emergency situations do not require prior consent
B. He or she must obtain written consent for invasive procedures
C. This is not a function of the LPN/LVN; the nurse should call his or her supervisor
D. The patient must be alert in order to obtain informed consent

ANS: A
Response: If the situation requires an immediate life-saving intervention, it does not require prior consent.
Chapter: Ethics and Law

3. Mr. B. is a 65-year-old attorney who has been admitted to your floor for blood work and neurological examinations. He is loud and verbally demanding of the staff. He says, "I know my rights. You nurses have to do whatever I ask. It's your job." The nurse responds:
A. "That is not one or your rights, Mr. B."
B. "You are taking time away from other patients, Mr. B."
C. "The Patient's Bill of Rights does make some provisions, Mr. B. Let me sit and talk with you about those rights."
D. "Why are you so angry, Mr. B?"
ANS: C
Response: This is the most therapeutic communication technique because it acknowledges the patient's concern, validates his idea of "his rights," and offers the nurse's time in assisting the patient.
Chapter: Ethics and Law

4. Marcy, a charge nurse on the floor, calls to say that she forgot to chart the 1400 dose of chlorpromazine (Thorazine) for Mrs. Fritz. She asks, "Please sign it for me. You saw me give it just before we counted the narcotics at the change of shift." The legal responsibility of the nurse is to:
A. Sign out psychoactive medications for other nurses because medications are so closely monitored
B. Forbid the LPN/LVN to administer psychoactive medications
C. Support the charge nurse's request, because this is a direct request from a supervisor
D. Require only the nurse who gives medications to sign for them
ANS: D
Response: Legal and ethical requirements for nurses state that each nurse must only sign or countersign for those interventions that he or she actually performs.
Chapter: Ethics and Law

5. Mr. Unsure is a 73-year-old man who is brought to the agency for treatment of second-degree burns. He answers questions clearly, but his daughter says, "Don't listen to him. He is confused and incompetent. I'm sure he has Alzheimer's disease, and I'm trying to get him committed. I will make medical decisions for him." The LPN/LVN caring for Mr. Unsure should:
A. Respect the rights of Mr. Unsure until he is legally determined to be "incompetent"
B. Tell Mr. Unsure that his daughter said he is incompetent
C. Alert the staff that Mr. Unsure's daughter is going to cause trouble
D. Call Mr. Unsure's son to see what he thinks about the situation
ANS: A
Response: Nurses are considered legally responsible if they do not perform according to the patient's wishes until such a time as that patient is legally determined to be "incompetent." Family wishes should be considered, but the patient is ultimately responsible until legal papers support otherwise.
Chapter: Ethics and Law

6. The main purpose of nursing regulations and standards of practice is to protect:
A. Nurses
B. Doctors
C. The public
D. The hospital
ANS: C
Response: Regulations on nursing practice are in place to protect the public, as well as to protect nurses; however, the main purpose is the safety and welfare of the people that nurses serve.
Chapter: Ethics and Law

7. A 30-year-old patient has a hypnotic ordered for bedtime, which is 2100 at your facility. Not wanting to commit a medication error, you strongly encourage him or her to take the medication, even though the patient states, "I never went to bed this early at home. I would prefer to take it in an hour." The patient cooperatively takes the medication

but awakens 3 hours later. He or she is disoriented and falls while crawling out of bed, resulting in a broken hip. The patient threatens to "sue that nurse!" Legally:
A. You are right to promote a stable medication schedule.
B. The patient's right to choose sleeping hours is a priority over hospital routines.
C. The doctor's order prevails.
D. The time of the medication administration should not have anything to do with the patient's confusion.
ANS: B
Response: The patient has a right to refuse or choose when to take sleep medication. If there are direct contraindications relating to the medication, the choice becomes a medical decision.
Chapter: Ethics and Law

8. Some states are adopting a set of patient's rights specifically for psychiatric patients. Which of the following might be included in these patients' rights?
A. The right to marry
B. The right to work/employment
C. The right to sue or be sued
D. All of the above
ANS: D
Response: All of the above. A person with mental illness has the right to maintain as much normalcy in their life as possible.
Chapter: Ethics and Law

9. The Community Mental Health Centers Act requires that communities offer some form of help around the clock to citizens in need. Which of the following would meet this requirement?
A. Women's shelter
B. Free-standing crisis center
C. Hospital
D. All of the above
ANS: D
Response: All of the above. Twenty-four-hour emergency rooms, trauma centers, crisis nurseries, and respite centers are other places that might provide care to people in need of mental health care.
Chapter: Ethics and Law

10. A nurse is preparing a 24-year-old female patient for her clinic appointment. When the nurse takes her vital signs, he or she notes discoloration on the woman's upper arm, shoulder, and neck and asks her how these areas became discolored. She sobs and tells the nurse about her abusive relationship and her reluctance to go to a shelter for fear of being found by her abuser. An appropriate response would be:
A. "Why are you afraid to go to the shelter?"
B. "I think it's a good idea. It's for your own safety."
C. "Locations of shelters are not published and the names of the people in the shelter are protected.
D. "Your abuser will not be able to find you if you are in a shelter."
ANS: C
Response: Shelters may advertise a phone number or even publish the address of the business office but the actual location of the residence is to be kept confidential. The other response options that the nurse offers are blocks to communication, such as using the word "why," and offering advice and false hope. An abuser may find out where the abused is sheltered from sources other than the shelter staff.
Chapter: Ethics and Law

Developmental Psychology

1. When caring for a young child, nurses realize that "trust" is part of normal growth and development. "Trust" is developed in which of the following age groups?
A. Infancy
B. Preschool
C. School age
D. Adolescence
ANS: A

138

Response: *Trust,* as defined by Erikson and others, is a response that is learned in infancy.
Chapter: Developmental Psychology

2. Language development is considered to be a learned behavior. Nurses encourage language development in infants and toddlers by:
A. Using "baby talk"
B. Talking to the infants as they would talk to adults
C. Using simple, age-appropriate words
D. Using full, long sentences
ANS: C
Response: Using simple, age-appropriate words creates honesty and promotes a child's understanding of language.
Chapter: Developmental Psychology

3. When teaching the parent(s) of a toddler, nurses discuss the dangers of aspiration that may be caused by small toys and other objects in the home. Toddlers are at risk for swallowing small objects because
A. They learn by experiencing objects orally
B. They know they will get attention if they put things in their mouths
C. They are purposely frightening their parent(s)
D. They are bored
ANS: A
Response: Children learn and gain knowledge by experiencing their environment in any way they can. This often involves using the mouth, which may place the child at risk for aspiration.
Chapter: Developmental Psychology

4. A young mother is crying and states that she is "a bad mother" because she has to leave her preschool-aged child at day care. Which of the following would be your therapeutic response to her?
A. "Oh, you'll get over that feeling in a few days."
B. "Lots of mothers do that. Why do you feel like a bad mother?"
C. "The people at day care are licensed. Your child is in good hands."
D. "It must be difficult to leave your child, but this may be a good opportunity for him or her to learn how to interact with peers."
ANS: D
Response: Your response implies what the mother might be experiencing and reinforces a positive effect of day care, without belittling the feelings of the mother. You also avoid focusing on the mother's act of crying.
Chapter: Developmental Psychology

5. Michael and Marcia are 13-year-old twins in the clinic with their parent who is concerned because Marcia is reaching puberty and Michael is not. Their parent is concerned about the difference in their sexual development. You are able to tell the parent:
A. "Both genders mature sexually at about the same time."
B. "Males generally mature 1 to 2 years before   females."
C. "Females generally mature 1 to 2 years before males."
D. "Females start to mature before males do but males usually reach sexual maturity before females."
ANS: C
Response: It is common for females to develop as much as 4 years ahead of males in this age group. The males will catch up in middle to late adolescence and, then, both genders will progress at approximately the same rate of development.
Chapter: Developmental Psychology

6. Tommy is 6-years-old and diabetic. When planning care with Tommy and his parent(s), you
A. Involve Tommy in decisions about his diet
B. Tell Tommy what he can and cannot eat
C. Tell his parents what "special" desserts and snacks are "good" for him
D. Tell Tommy that he is "different" from his friends
ANS: A

Response: Involving any patient, children included, in decisions about their treatment will help to increase compliance and knowledge about the plan of care.
Chapter: Developmental Psychology

7. A major cause of rebellious behavior in children and adolescents is:
A. Setting fair and consistent boundaries
B. Feeling rejection or indifference from their parents
C. Expecting age-appropriate responsibility
D. Spending 1 hour daily in "family time"
ANS: B
Response: Adolescents need to know that they are being listened to and valued as individuals. Indifference or rejection by parents or persons they look up to is interpreted by the adolescent as he or she having little or no value in that adult's life. The adolescent will rebel as a way of making his or her needs known.
Chapter: Developmental Psychology

8. Your 78-year-old patient who has been admitted S/P cerebrovascular accident has suffered a right visual field loss. The patient is alert and follows commands well. You are concerned about the patient's self-esteem, as well as meeting his or her safety and physical needs. Your most therapeutic intervention for this patient would be:
A. Approach the patient from his or her affected side
B. Approach the patient from his or her unaffected side
C. Place utensils and items the patient uses on his or her unaffected side
D. Frequently encourage the patient to position him or herself so he or she can scan the environment
ANS: D
Response: This choice not only keeps the patient as independent as possible, but it teaches and reinforces the patient's need to be aware of one's environment, in order to maintain safety, mobility, and other activities required in daily life.
Chapter: Developmental Psychology

9. Mrs. Greene, who is 68-years-old, is at your clinic for her annual physical. She is quiet and does not use her usual quick sense of humor. She tells you, "I feel like an old rag. I can't hear or see as well as I could before. What's wrong with me?" You are able to tell her:
A. "Mrs. Greene, some vision and hearing loss is normal in the aging process. The doctor can run some tests and discuss options with you."
B. "Mrs. Greene, don't worry. I'm sure it's nothing!"
C. "Well, at least you don't need to worry about driving anymore."
D. "Why are you feeling so concerned, Mrs. Greene?"
ANS: A
Response: You have informed the patient without belittling her concerns. The information that you have provided her with will allow the doctor and the patient to discuss further testing possibilities.

10. Mr. and Mrs. Close are a happily married couple in their 70s who have been together for 50 years. They present together at your clinic and seem reluctant to state their concern. In response to your observation about their uneasiness, Mr. Close tells you that they have been having difficulties with intercourse and don't know who to talk to. "Our children think it is shameful that we still have sex at our ages, so we can't talk to them." You respond:
A. "I think your children have your best interest at heart."
B. "What do you think about people your age being sexual?"
C. "It is perfectly normal to be intimate at any age. Here are some pamphlets about sexuality in later adult years."
D. "I wish more people thought as you do about sexuality!"
ANS: C
Response: You have provided information to this couple in a factual and nonjudgmental manner.
Chapter: Developmental Psychology

11. Johnny is a 5-year-old child who is on your medical floor for treatment of an exacerbation of his leukemia. His family lives a long distance away. You see him sitting alone and he says he is "too tired and sad to play with the other children." Your therapeutic intervention for Johnny would be:

A. "Johnny, I have some time now and I'd like to play with you. What shall we do?"
B. "Johnny, you know it won't do you any good to feel sad."
C. "Johnny, playing with the other children might help you to forget that your family is not here."
D. "Johnny, you should be in bed if you are so tired."
ANS: A
Response: You have sensed Johnny's sadness about missing his family. Your response shows Johnny that the nurse is paying attention to him, that he has special needs, and that he is allowed to make some decisions about what activities he might enjoy.
Chapter: Developmental Psychology

12. You are caring for a 5-year-old child who has pneumonia. You bring the child's dinner tray to the room and the child says, "I can't feed myself. I'm sick." You respond:
A. "If you don't eat, you can't go home!"
B. "If you wait for 10 minutes, I'll be back to help you."
C. "At least try to eat what you can."
D. "Your roommate does not need anyone to feed him or her and he or she is younger than you are!"
ANS: B
Response: Usually giving a child a few minutes will stimulate him or her to self-feed. By choosing this response, you allow the child some control, independent decision making, and have also been attentive to the emotional needs of the child.
Chapter: Developmental Psychology

13. You notice a 7-year-old child who has begun thumb sucking during an extended hospitalization. According to the parents, this was not part of the child's usual behavior prior to hospitalization. Your response is:
A. Offer to color with the child as a diversion.
B. Report this behavior to the child's doctor.
C. Tell the child that "only babies suck their thumbs."
D. Allow the thumb sucking and say nothing to the child.
ANS: D
Response: The child is demonstrating regression, which is normal for a child when he or she is stressed. Regression helps reduce the child's anxiety. Diversion may be helpful later but at this time it may actually increase the child's anxiety.
Chapter: Developmental Psychology

14. You are caring for a 6-month-old infant who has been hospitalized since birth for congenital defects. You would expect all of the following in an infant who has been in the hospital for this period of time *except*:
A. Slower than normal weight gain
B. Focusing on objects rather than the face of the caregiver
C. Excessive crying
D. Limited emotional responses
ANS: C
Response: Excessive crying would be consistent with an infant who has learned "basic trust" and expects someone to attend to his or her needs. This type of behavior is not consistent with an infant who has been deprived of consistent parental care or prolonged hospitalization.
Chapter: Developmental Psychology

15. The primary reason for rebellious behavior in adolescents is:
A. Parents who are indifferent toward the children
B. Parents who set limits on the curfew
C. Parents who provide an allowance in exchange for the responsibilities a child has at home
D. Parents who insist on a daily family meal
ANS: A
Response: Parents who are indifferent or appear to reject their adolescent children, for reasons of employment or anything else, give the adolescent the opportunity to start living by his or her own rules or the rules of the peer group. Parents who then attempt to intervene or become involved will give the impression of mistrusting and invalidating their adolescent; thus, adding to the adolescent's rebellious behavior.
Chapter: Developmental Psychology

16. You are the nurse assigned to teach a class for first-time parents. They express concern and nervousness about sudden infant death syndrome (SIDS) and how to keep their babies safe. You tell the parents that the safest way to position their newborn when he or she is sleeping is to lay the baby on its
A. Back with its head flat
B. Abdomen with its head slightly elevated
C. Side with its head flat
D. Back with its head slightly elevated
ANS: C
Response: The safest way to prevent breathing problems is to lay the baby flat on its back or on either one of its sides.
Chapter: Developmental Psychology

17. You are caring for a 16-year-old male who was hurt when he fell from a personal watercraft. He has refused to perform his physical therapy and has now developed contractures in his arms and legs. He still continues to resist therapy. Your nursing interventions for this patient would include:
A. Asking his friends to convince him to worked harder
B. Allowing the patient to make decisions related to his care
C. Telling him that he will only worsen his pain by not cooperating with therapy
D. Setting strict limits on this patient's behavior
ANS: B
Response: Adolescents need to feel independence and control of their situation. Allowing these increases the probability that the adolescent will cooperate with care. If you allow the adolescent to be more actively involved you will validate his or her need to feel that adults take him or her seriously.
Chapter: Developmental Psychology

18. Five-year-old William is present in the room when his father passes away. He is aware that his mother and grandparents are crying, but he tells them not to worry. "This happens all the time on my cartoon show. Come on, Daddy; wake up now." Nurses understand that children also experience the stages of grief. As the nurse caring for this family, you know that at William's age it is important to:
A. Divert William's attention away from his father by asking about his favorite cartoon show
B. Tell William that this is not his fault and he did nothing to cause his father's death
C. Ask another relative to take William home
D. Reassure William that his mother will explain the situation to him later
ANS: B
Response: Children in this age group need to know the death was not their fault. It is important to keep them feeling involved, safe, and secure. Honesty that they can understand is important.
Chapter: Developmental Psychology

19. A parent with a 2-year-old child comes to the clinic as a walk-in. They had been cooking on the outdoor grill when the parent turned away for a second and the child touched the grill, receiving burns to the hands. Given the age of the child, the appropriate statement from the parent would be:
A. "We will not leave the grill unattended when the children are near."
B. "I guess we just won't use the grill until the children are older."
C. "It was not my fault. I just looked away for a second."
D. "I guess the child has learned what the word 'hot' means now."
ANS: A
Response: Response "A" is the response that is actually age appropriate for the safety of the child. This response also shows responsible parenting on the part of the adult.
Chapter: Developmental Psychology

Mental Health: Sociocultural Influences

1. A distraught young father has brought his 3-year-old daughter to the clinic. She is ill and showing symptoms of pneumonia. As you take the history, the father tells you his wife was recently killed in a traffic accident. "How will I

ever raise my daughter right? A girl needs her mother!" A truth about parenting that the nurse can share with the father is:

A. The child will do better with both a mother and a father.
B. Parenting is stressful and parents of either gender need "adult" time for themselves.
C. The child will receive adequate female role modeling at day care; the father need not be concerned.
D. All of the above.

ANS: B

Response: Parents need to take time for themselves to maintain a healthy lifestyle but are concerned that their children may or may not get appropriate role modeling. It has been demonstrated that both genders can be successful at parenting and a single parent can be just as effective as a traditional two-parent family.

Chapter: Mental Health: Sociocultural Influences

2. A discussion among nurses during lunch centers on the correlation between socioeconomic status and the incidence of abnormal behavior. From your study of psychology, you remember at least one study that showed:

A. No correlation between socioeconomic status and abnormal behavior
B. The higher one's socioeconomic status, the lower the incidence of abnormal behavior
C. The lower the socioeconomic status, the higher the incidence of abnormal behavior
D. The lower the socioeconomic status, the lower the incidence of abnormal behavior

ANS: C

Response: Answer "C" refers to the Eron and Peterson study. It is important for nurses to remember that these are generalizations and do not hold true in every situation or every type of abnormal behavior. For example, the reference cited in this question is truer for patients with schizophrenia than it is for patients with mood disorders.

Chapter: Mental Health: Sociocultural Influences

Coping and Defense Mechanisms

1. *Regression* is best defined as:

A. A retreat to a less stressful time in the one's life
B. An immature response technique
C. An assertive response
D. A therapeutic mechanism

ANS: A

Response: Regression provides the "security" the patient felt during a safer and less stressful period in his or her life.

Chapter: Coping and Defense Mechanisms

2. One of your patients has just received a diagnosis of terminal cancer. You go to speak with the patient and find him or her talking on the phone. The patient sees you and laughingly responds, "What are you all so concerned about? The tests were obviously wrong. I'm not that sick!" He or she is displaying:

A. Transference
B. Regression
C. Denial
D. Identification

ANS: C

Response: "Denial" is the unconscious refusal to accept situations as they are. (It is also one of the stages of grief.)

Chapter: Coping and Defense Mechanisms

3. A patient who has survived a motor vehicle accident has just learned that the passenger in the car has died. The police are attempting to obtain information from the "survivor," but the patient is unable to recall even being in the car. The nurse on duty realizes this is:

A. Dissociation
B. Denial
C. Regression
D. Transference

ANS: A

Response: The patient has temporarily separated or "divorced" the painful situation from the consciousness.

Chapter: Coping and Defense Mechanisms

4. Peptic ulcers, headaches, and other disorders may be an expression of emotional disturbance. Nurses know that this is identified as:
A. Hypochondriasis
B. Repression
C. Conversion
D. Splitting
ANS: C
Response: In conversion or conversion disorder, the patient "converts" emotional stress into physical symptoms.
Chapter: Coping and Defense Mechanisms

5. Mark and Julie have been married for 5 years. Julie is very attractive and has recently had an affair with a neighbor. She is jealous of Mark and his career and frequently accuses him of "running around." Julie is demonstrating:
A. Identification
B. Reaction formation
C. Denial
D. Projection/scapegoatism
ANS: D
Response: Julie is unconsciously displacing her guilt on Mark and his career.
Chapter: Coping and Defense Mechanisms

6. Anisha, who is 3-years-old, is an only child. She was completely toilet trained 6 months ago. She has recently started to attend day care, and she has begun wetting herself. Her mother is concerned and you tell her that Anisha is most likely experiencing:
A. Regression
B. Repression
C. Manipulation
D. Compensation
ANS: A
Response: Anisha is most likely expressing her emotional upset over starting day care by retreating to a time when she was more secure; thus, she has begun wetting herself since it was part of that time.
Chapter: Coping and Defense Mechanisms

7. A male college student who is overweight and unable to participate in competitive sports becomes the life of the party and starts driving a popular sports car. He is displaying:
A. Compensation
B. Reaction formation
C. Transference
D. Identification
ANS: A
Response: "Compensation" is the defense mechanism through which the student attempts to increase his self-esteem by excelling in one area to unconsciously make up for a real or imagined defect in another area.
Chapter: Coping and Defense Mechanisms

8. When people express anxiety through physical symptoms, they are experiencing:
A. Compensation
B. Conversion
C. Regression
D. Introjection
ANS: B
Response: "Conversion" or "conversion reaction" is the defense mechanism of expressing anxiety by unconsciously "converting" it into physical symptoms.
Chapter: Coping and Defense Mechanisms

9. You have been working with a female patient who has delusions of persecution and who hears "voices" sometimes. She has also attempted to poison her boyfriend after a fight. You greet her and ask her how she is. She says to you, "She's a bad person!" She is exhibiting:
A. Denial
B. Transference
C. Regression
D. Dissociation
ANS: D
Response: The patient is exhibiting "dissociation." She has separated herself from the emotional trauma of the attempt on her boyfriend's life by speaking as though she is someone else.
Chapter: Coping and Defense Mechanisms

10. Maria was a victim of sexual abuse as a young child. She is improving with therapy and is now able to recall some of these abusive events. Maria was exhibiting:
A. Denial
B. Repression
C. Regression
D. Rationalization
ANS: B
Response: Maria has repressed or "stuffed" the pain of the sexual abuse into her unconscious. There is no indication at this point that she had dissociated the events.
Chapter: Coping and Defense Mechanisms

11. Patients who unconsciously refuse to accept a situation as it truly is display:
A. Confabulation
B. Lying
C. Denial
D. Identification
ANS: C
Response: "Denial" is the unconscious defense mechanism of refusing to accept situations as they actually are. "Lying" is a conscious activity.
Chapter: Coping and Defense Mechanisms

12. A patient is scheduled for major surgery tomorrow morning. You ask the patient if he or she has any questions about the surgery. The patient says "no" and then proceeds to tell you about the activity in the stock market that day. You believe that this patient is displaying:
A. Denial
B. Transference
C. Regression
D. Splitting
ANS: A
Response: The patient is unconsciously refusing to deal with the upcoming surgery.
Chapter: Coping and Defense Mechanisms

13. Dave is a 32-year-old man who portrays himself as an individual with high moral standards. He is a member of a strict religious group and he is very judgmental of others. Dave is brought to your hospital to be treated for wounds sustained when he "allegedly" attempted to rape a neighbor. As his nurse, you know that the defense mechanism Dave portrays in the alleged rape is:
A. Denial
B. Repression
C. Compensation
D. Reaction formation
ANS: D
Response: "Reaction formation" or "overcompensation" is behavior that is the exact opposite of the usual behavior. There is also a conflict between the id and the superego in this type of behavior.
Chapter: Coping and Defense Mechanisms

14. You are getting ready for work when you see your 4-year-old imitating your actions (i.e., shaving, brushing teeth, and etc.). Your 4-year-old is exhibiting a form of:
A. Identification
B. Compensation
C. Regression
D. Reaction formation
ANS: A
Response: This 4-year-old is exhibiting a form of "identification." The child is "role-modeling" the actions of the person he or she admires.
Chapter: Coping and Defense Mechanisms

15. Your charge nurse has been in a meeting with the director of nursing (DON). The DON has been given some very unpleasant mandates by the administrator and has very abruptly handed them down to the DON who has, in turn, forcefully handed them down to the charge nurse. It is now the charge nurse's task to hand them down to the nursing staff. The charge nurse gives the news to the staff in a very angry manner. This procession of behavior throughout the nursing hierarchy is an example of:
A. Sublimation
B. Identification
C. Transference
D. Reaction formation
ANS: C
Response: This is an example of "transference." People who demonstrate this defense mechanism take their anxiety out on people or objects that they perceive to be less powerful than they are.
Chapter: Coping and Defense Mechanisms

16. Marlene has just finalized a painful divorce; she lost her home and many of her possessions in the settlement. She now spends most of the day imagining herself living with her favorite movie star in a mansion on the beach, with unlimited wealth and love. Marlene is experiencing:
A. Compensation
B. Denial
C. Regression
D. Fantasy/escapism
ANS: D
Response: This is an example of fantasy/escapism. Marlene is using imagery and "wishful thinking," but she is using it as an unconscious escape from her reality.
Chapter: Coping and Defense Mechanisms

17. Susie is 5-years-old. She has been toilet trained for 3 years. She has just started preschool and has never been away from her parents. Recently, Susie has begun wetting herself during the day and at night. Susie is experiencing:
A. Repression
B. Regression
C. Reaction formation
D. Retribution
ANS: B
Response: Susie is expressing a response to the anxiety of preschool. She has retreated to a time that was less emotionally stressful and is displaying some of those behaviors, including incontinence.
Chapter: Coping and Defense Mechanisms

18. The defense mechanism that unconsciously allows pent-up emotions to be directed at someone or something that is less stressful than the primary source of the anxiety is:
A. Compensation
B. Identification
C. Repression
D. Displacement

ANS: D
Response: "Displacement" or "transference" is the unconscious mechanism of directing anxiety at someone or something that is perceived as less threatening than the root of the anxiety.
Chapter: Coping and Defense Mechanisms

19. The associate nurse in the local junior high school sees a group of students wearing identical T-shirts depicting a popular WWF wrestler. The principal has told the students the message is not appropriate for school apparel. The nurse recognizes the choice of clothing as a possible example of:
A. Compensation
B. Identification
C. Repression
D. Conversion
ANS: B
Response: Identification is displayed.
Chapter: Coping and Defense Mechanisms

20. A client has just been physically abused by his or her partner. He or she is in the examining room crying softly, rocking, and sucking his or her thumb. The nurse identifies this behavior as possible:
A. Compensation
B. Intellectualization
C. Regression
D. Denial
ANS: C
Response: The patient is exhibiting behaviors indicative of a less stressful period in one's life (in this case, childhood).
Chapter: Coping and Defense Mechanisms

21. Jerome is a young adult who is admitted to your medical unit for possible alcohol poisoning. He has an IV for hydration and has been in and out of consciousness. His wife has just arrived. He awakens, notices the IV, and sees the nurse speaking with his wife. Jerome pulls out his IV, attempts to get out of bed, and begins shouting, "Get me out of here. I am just fine. I don't belong in this place!" The nurse realizes this behavior is an example of:
A. Compensation
B. Intellectualization
C. Regression
D. Denial
ANS: D
Response: The patient is displaying "denial." Because of the patient's diagnosis, his behavior could also be secondary to his alcohol poisoning, and may include fear, hallucination, anger or any number of responses associated with alcohol overuse and poisoning.
Chapter: Coping and Defense Mechanisms

Treating Mental Health Alterations

1. The main goal of the therapeutic milieu is:
A. Make the patient feel "at home."
B. Manipulate the patient into behaving appropriately.
C. Encourage the client to relate more effectively with others.
D. Allow the staff to control the patient.
ANS: C
Response: Relating effectively with others helps to increase self-esteem, which will allow the patient to deal with daily interpersonal situations.
Chapter: Treating Mental Health Alterations

2. The most effective intervention for a confused patient in the therapeutic environment is:
A. Develop a trusting nurse-patient relationship.

B. Adhere to a strict routine.
C. Provide many activities for the patient to choose from.
D. Involve patient in group activities.
ANS: A
Response: Developing a trusting relationship helps the patient to learn to trust in other situations, become self-responsible, and become more involved in his or her daily activities.
Chapter: Treating Mental Health Alterations

3. When helping to intervene in a crisis situation, it is important for nurses to:
A. Do everything that the patient in crisis requests
B. Assure the patient that everything will be fine if he or she just calms down
C. Place the person in four-point restraints
D. Honestly reinforce the patient's strengths and abilities
ANS: D
Response: Focusing on a patient's strengths helps him or her to regain some control of the situation and to put the problem into a more manageable perspective.
Chapter: Treating Mental Health Alterations

4. Nurses understand that there is a mind-body connection; therefore, the nurse knows that the system most closely related to the "fight or flight" response in physical or emotional crises is the
A. Central nervous system
B. Sympathetic nervous system
C. Peripheral nervous system
D. Parasympathetic nervous system
ANS: B
Response: The sympathetic nervous system releases epinephrine, which increases pulse, increases oxygen supply to the muscles, and constricts peripheral vessels.
Chapter: Treating Mental Health Alterations

5. You are on duty when Mr. Jones is admitted at 0300. Mr. Jones is a 42-year-old male patient with schizophrenia. He has been hospitalized multiple times for his schizophrenia because he says he "feels better" and he does not take his medications. A long-acting medication that can be given IM, which you suggest to the physician is:
A. Prolixin decanoate
B. Mellaril
C. Melatonin
D. Lithium decanoate
ANS: A
Response: Prolixin decanoate can be given on an average of every 2 weeks. This drug increases compliance, while keeping the symptoms under control; thus, it allows the patient to lead a more natural life in his or her community.
Chapter: Treating Mental Health Alterations

6. Lithium carbonate is ordered for a new patient on your floor. You know that Lithium carbonate is the drug of choice for:
A. Schizophrenia
B. Major depression
C. Bulimia
D. Bipolar depression
ANS: D
Response: Lithium carbonate is the drug of choice for controlling the symptoms, especially manic episodes, of bipolar depression.
Chapter: Treating Mental Health Alterations

7. An important aspect of patient teaching for a person taking lithium carbonate is:
A. "It is important to have your blood level checked when your doctor orders it."
B. "You should stop taking all other medication for 2 weeks."

C. "It is required to administer a daily glucose test on your urine."
D. "Lithium is a salt, so be sure that you do not add salt to your food."
ANS: A
Response: It is important for the patient to monitor the electrolyte balance in the blood because lithium is a salt. Lithium's effects can alter electrolyte balance, so it is important that the lithium level is carefully monitored.
Chapter: Treating Mental Health Alterations

8. Drugs such as trihexyphenidyl (Artane) or benztropine (Cogentin) are often prescribed to be used with:
A. Antianxiety drugs/minor tranquilizers
B. Antipsychotic drugs/major tranquilizers
C. Tricyclic antidepressants
D. Stimulants
ANS: B
Response: These "antiparkinson agents" are used to counteract the extrapyramidal side effects of the antipsychotic drugs.
Chapter: Treating Mental Health Alterations

9. Sally Sad will begin electroconvulsive therapy (ECT) in 1 week. Which of the following physician orders would a nurse expect to see?
A. "Take NPO after ECT treatments."
B. "Discontinue all psychotropic medications 3 days prior to ECT treatment."
C. "Do not medicate the patient prior to ECT treatment."
D. "Administer 100 mg of succinylcholine 30 minutes before ECT."
ANS: B
Response: It is customary to stop psychotropic medications prior to ECT. Patients may resume psychotropic medications after treatment if the doctor chooses.
Chapter: Treating Mental Health Alterations

10. When a patient's coping mechanisms no longer work to control anxiety, nurses know the patient may next experience:
A. Mental illness
B. Suicide
C. A crisis situation
D. Euphoria
ANS: C
Response: Crisis is generally the next state a person will experience when coping mechanisms are no longer effective in "handling" their anxiety. (The other above options may also occur as the crisis worsens.)
Chapter: Treating Mental Health Alterations

11. Patient A is taking an antianxiety medication. You know you should be most concerned about which of the following effects?
A. Hypertension
B. Extrapyramidal side effects
C. Polyuria
D. Physical/psychological dependence
ANS: D
Response: The main concern for people taking antianxiety medication is the potential for either physical or psychological dependence.
Chapter: Treating Mental Health Alterations

12. You do the intake assessment on a young female patient in the clinic and you notice hand tremors. Her chart indicates that she started on chlorpromazine (Thorazine) following her last visit 2 weeks ago. Your first action is:
A. Report the symptom to the doctor immediately.
B. Teach her finger-strengthening exercises.

C. Tell her to stop taking the medication immediately.

D. Inform her that "this happens" and "not to worry."

ANS: A

Response: It is your responsibility, as the nurse, to inform the physician of any side effects of the medication. Only the doctor will decide on changes in the patient's treatment.

Chapter: Treating Mental Health Alterations

13. Patricia is a 32-year-old patient who has been taking a monoamine oxidase (MAO) inhibitor for 1 month. She arrives for her examination, and she excitedly shares with you that she has a date for a wine and cheese party this evening with a brand new boyfriend. You carefully tell her:

A. "Sounds like fun! I wish I was going!"

B. "Remember that wine and cheese are two foods that you are cautioned against on your medication."

C. "How exciting! What is the occasion?"

D. "You know you shouldn't drink alcohol when you are taking psychotropic medications!"

ANS: B

Response: Wine and cheese are two foods that contain tyramine and should be avoided when taking MAO inhibitors.

Chapter: Treating Mental Health Alterations

14. Bob is a 24-year-old patient with schizophrenia who lives in a group home. Bob presents at the clinic with bad sunburn. He tells you he "went to the beach with the others at the home." You look at Bob's list of medications and remind him that photosensitivity is a side effect of his

A. Lithium carbonate

B. Prozac

C. Mellaril

D. Thorazine

ANS: D

Response: Of the four medications listed, photosensitivity is a frequently occurring side effect of Thorazine. Patients who take Thorazine may experience severe sunburn if they are not adequately covered when exposed to the sun.

Chapter: Treating Mental Health Alterations

15. A woman enters the emergency room and begs the nurses to "help" her. As the nurse assisting her, your first assessment would be:

A. "From your perspective, please explain what happened to you."

B. "Has this ever happened to you or any of your other family members before?"

C. "What is it that you want us to do for you?"

D. "Would you like me to call your parents?"

ANS: A

Response: Response "A" shows that you are interested in the patient's perspective and that you have no preconceived ideas about the patient or her situation.

Chapter: Treating Mental Health Alterations

16. A group of adolescents run into your clinic, dragging one of their friends. They tell you, "He tried to kill himself." Which of the following interventions is the best option for the nurse to use with a suicidal teenager?

A. Tell the adolescent that this is no way to gain the respect of an adult.

B. Tell the adolescent how to cope with his/her situation.

C. Explore with the adolescent options other than suicide to help his or her situation.

D. Tell the adolescent, "Nothing can be that bad!"

ANS: C

Response: Exploring options with the adolescent shows concern for the individual, as well as value for his or her opinions. Keeping the adolescent involved in his or her treatment plan will increase his or her responsibility and compliance with the plan.

Chapter: Treating Mental Health Alterations

17. Which of the following people would a nurse recognize as at the highest risk for suicide?

A. A patient with a well-organized plan
B. A patient who has friends or family who have attempted suicide
C. A patient who is in a deep depression
D. A patient has a strong support system
ANS: A
Response: The patient who has an organized plan and intends to carry it out is at highest risk for suicide. Patients who are deeply depressed do not usually have the energy to plan and carry out a suicide, although they may contemplate it.
Chapter: Treating Mental Health Alterations

18. Keesha, a 33-year-old patient, presents at the clinic for a work-related injury. She is not specific about the injury, but does repeatedly state she thinks her supervisor "doesn't like" her and that she feels "picked on." She says she is "depressed" at work and she wants to know about a new "herbal" medication called SAMe. She said she heard it is "completely safe" and asks what you think. Your best response to Keesha would be:
A. "I've heard that too. Go ahead and try it."
B. "I don't have enough information. Please ask the doctor during your examination."
C. "I think those things are very dangerous."
D. "I wouldn't take it, if I were you."
ANS: B
Response: Your statement provides a basic therapeutic communication skill and it is legally correct statement. Nurses encourage patients to ask similar questions of their physicians. The other choices block therapeutic communication.
Chapter: Treating Mental Health Alterations

19. Community health is evolving. Now, licensed practical nurses/licensed vocational nurses (LPNs/LVNs) have opportunities to serve the community in ways that have not previously been available to them. Some community health nursing involves special credentialing; some does not. One way an LPN/LVN may be able to assist people in the community who have mental health conditions is as a(n):
A. Occupational health nurse
B. Public health nurse
C. Nurse practitioner
D. Parish nurse
ANS: D
Response: Parish nursing may, depending on the requirements of the faith community, be an option for the LPN/LVN wishing to assist with health issues (including issues of mental health). The positions may be volunteer but will offer helpful services to those in the community, as well as provide valuable experience for the LPN/LVN. The other choices usually require a minimum of a registered nurse licensure and further certification.
Chapter: Treating Mental Health Alterations

Mental Health Alterations

1. A 40-year-old patient arrives at the clinic. Crying, she says, "I just don't feel well. I think the doctors think I'm faking it. They just keep asking me questions and taking blood. Why don't they give me something to help?" Which of the following is the best response by the licensed practical nurse/licensed vocational nurse (LPN/LVN)?
A. "It must be very frustrating to constantly feel ill."
B. "The doctors take blood to check for certain illnesses that might be causing your symptoms."
C. "It is important that you share these concerns with your doctor."
D. All of the above
ANS: D
Response: All of these responses are examples of therapeutic communication that may assist the patient with her concerns.
Chapter: Mental Health Alterations

2. In cases that are similar to the case above, nurses know that:
A. Physical and mental conditions may be easily differentiated
B. Electrolyte imbalances may cause behaviors that are also seen in people who have mental illnesses

C. Blood work will not show possible reasons for mental health symptoms
D. There is seldom a correlation between mental and physical health
ANS: B
Response: Blood work that reflects electrolyte imbalances and nutritional imbalances may be an indicator of behaviors that mimic mental illness. These imbalances may, in fact, be a causative factor in some mental illnesses. The mind-body connection in health is very important. It is not often easy to differentiate between mental and physical conditions because of the mind-body connection.
Chapter: Mental Health Alterations

Anxiety Disorders

1. Mrs. B has an irrational fear of elevators. In order to go to her testing in radiology, she must travel down floors. She is "partial weight bearing for bathroom privileges only." Your best nursing intervention for her is:
A. Demand that she use the elevator to combat the fear
B. Allow her to use the stairs and accompany her
C. Offer her a reward for using the elevator
D. Deny her pass privileges until she demonstrates ability to use the elevator
ANS: B
Response: Forcing her to ride the elevator at this time may only heighten the phobia to the point of panic.
Chapter: Anxiety Disorders

2. Nurses understand that an individual may demonstrate anxiety in all of the following ways *except*:
A. Antisocial behavior
B. Conversion
C. Identification
D. Displacement
ANS: A
Response: Antisocial behavior is more accurately associated with personality disorders than anxiety disorders.
Chapter: Anxiety Disorders

3. Which of the following would be the best nursing diagnosis for a patient with a phobia?
A. Anxiety related to (specific fear)
B. Knowledge deficit related to (specific fear)
C. Social isolation related to (specific fear)
D. Ineffective individual coping related to (specific fear)
ANS: D
Response: The patient with a phobic disorder most often has poor coping skills and is unable to process information relating to the fear.
Chapter: Anxiety Disorders

4. When doing a complete assessment on a patient with a phobia, the nurse would expect which of the following physical manifestations of anxiety?
A. Constricted pupils, increased heart rate, and peripheral vasodilation
B. Constricted pupils, hypoglycemia, and decreased heart rate
C. Dilated pupils, increased heart rate, and peripheral vasoconstriction
D. Dilated pupils, decreased heart rate, and vasodilation
ANS: C
Response: These manifestations are consistent with the sympathetic nervous system and associated with the "fight or flight" response.
Chapter: Anxiety Disorders

5. A nurse can assist a patient who is trying to decrease anxiety by:
A. Teaching the patient systematic desensitization
B. Modeling skills that assist in facing stressful situations

C. Teaching the patient to simply avoid the unpleasant situation
D. Instructing the patient that fear can be exciting
ANS: B
Response: Learning to use a variety of skills is a helpful tool for preventing or lessening stress in the patient's life.
Chapter: Anxiety Disorders

6. A parent presents at the clinic with a 4-year-old child. The child is crying and pacing. The parent states, "I can't take this any more," and leaves the child alone with you. You see in the child's chart that he or she has an anxiety disorder. Your best immediate nursing intervention is:
A. Remain there, in close contact with the child
B. Ask the child what the problem is
C. Tell the child to "be quiet; other patients are complaining"
D. Divert the child's attention to a game or toy
ANS: A
Response: Staying physically close to the child conveys a caring attitude, especially because the parent has left the child alone.
Chapter: Anxiety Disorders

7. A general nursing action to help minimize a patient's psychological stress is:
A. Give detailed explanations of the plan of care.
B. Inform the client that you are in charge of the situation and that there is no need to worry.
C. Learn what is important and of concern to the patient.
D. Discourage the patient from discussing unpleasant topics in order to decrease stress.
ANS: C
Response: Learning about the patient's concerns conveys the nurse's support and the nurse's care for the well-being of the patient.
Chapter: Anxiety Disorders

8. Which of the following statements is typical of a patient with generalized anxiety disorder?
A. The patient states they "must have medication to control their stress."
B. The state they "worry about things all the time."
C. The patient only experiences "signal anxiety."
D. The patient states feelings of hopelessness.
ANS: B
Response: It is very common for people with generalized anxiety disorder to worry about everything.
Chapter: Anxiety Disorders

9. While working with a woman who is experiencing post-traumatic stress disorder (PTSD) following a rape, the focus of your therapeutic nursing technique should be to help the patient to:
A. Begin legal action against the rapist
B. Repress the situation and move on with her life
C. See that allowing the situation to dominate her is not helping
D. Put the situation into perspective and understand what happened to her
ANS: D
Response: It is important for the patient to get on with her life, but she must first put the situation into perspective.
Chapter: Anxiety Disorders

10. The main goal set forth by the nurse for a patient experiencing PTSD is to:
A. Encourage the patient to describe the situation that led to the PTSD
B. Tell the patient that the danger is all over
C. Have the patient tell you what he or she should expect when he or she is about to have a flashback
D. Ensure that the patient gets 6 to 8 hours of uninterrupted sleep nightly
ANS: A
Response: Option "A" demonstrates the patient's knowledge and perspective about the incident.
Chapter: Anxiety Disorders

11. Discharge teaching for patients with anxiety disorders includes the information that *anxiety* can be described as:
A. A severe response to stress that only a few people ever experience
B. A conscious response
C. A behavior pattern that many people experience at one time or another
D. Unexplainable
ANS: C
Response: Anxiety is a common human experience, which involves physical and emotional responses when an individual is in a stressful situation.
Chapter: Anxiety Disorders

12. A 21-year-old male patient refuses to touch the silverware on his tray unless he holds them in a napkin. He believes all of the silverware is contaminated. When working with this patient, the nurse should:
A. Provide napkins for the patient
B. Refuse to provide napkins, because this is just a part of the illness and totally unnecessary
C. Use systematic desensitization
D. Provide the patient with a tour of the area where the dishes are sanitized
ANS: A
Response: The patient's ritual of holding the silverware in a napkin is a mechanism for decreasing his anxiety. The nurse should provide the patient with napkins until he learns to confront the anxiety when he is in therapy.
Chapter: Anxiety Disorders

13. Compulsions such as washing one's hands repeatedly or constantly checking doors to be sure they are locked develop because the patients are:
A. Consciously attempting to punish themselves or others
B. Responding to "the voices" telling them to perform the ritual
C. Unconsciously controlling unpleasant thoughts or feelings
D. Unaware that they are performing the ritual
ANS: C
Response: This is an unconscious response, which helps to divert and control the unpleasant thought or feeling and prevent one from acting on these.
Chapter: Anxiety Disorders

14. When collaborating on a care plan for a patient who has obsessive-compulsive disorder (OCD), nurses would do all of the following *except*:
A. Teach the patient about the nature of the disorder
B. Involve the client in the plan of care
C. Maintain a nonjudgmental atmosphere
D. Allow the ritual three times a day
ANS: D
Response: Setting a frequency limit on the behavior is unrealistic, sends the message that the ritual is acceptable "sometimes," and will only add to the patient's anxiety by denying the behavior that is supposed to decrease the anxiety.
Chapter: Anxiety Disorders

15. A patient in your medical unit is experiencing dyspnea. You also sense that the patient is anxious. As the nurse caring for this patient, you
A. Ignore the anxiety, because it will probably go away when the patient is breathing better
B. Notify the doctor
C. Reassure the patient that this is only temporary
D. Remain with the patient and be supportive of the situation
ANS: D
Response: Difficulty breathing can be very frightening and anxiety is common with dyspnea, so it is best to stay with the patient and calmly offer support.
Chapter: Anxiety Disorders

16. The nurse caring for a patient with PTSD knows that the etiology for this disorder is usually:
A. An unexpected life-threatening or catastrophic event
B. Any event that causes untoward anxiety
C. Ineffective coping capacity
D. Denial
ANS: A
Response: PTSD is a typical response to a severe anxiety-producing event that is not anticipated, such as a rape or a natural disaster.
Chapter: Anxiety Disorders

17. A patient presents at the walk-in clinic in extreme fear. The nurse knows that phobia rarely occurs unless that patient
A. Thinks about the feared object or situation
B. Talks about the feared object or situation
C. Realizes that the fear is not rational
D. Comes in contact with the feared object or situation
ANS: D
Response: Patients with phobias usually realize that the fear exists and that it is out of proportion. They generally have no phobic response unless they come in direct contact with the object or situation that produces the fear.
Chapter: Anxiety Disorders

18. A patient describes his or her periods of anxiety as "just horrible" and says that he or she "never knows when it's going to happen." The patient tells you, "I feel like I can't breathe." You realize that the patient's complaints are common symptoms of:
A. Phobia
B. Panic disorder
C. PTSD
D. Mania
ANS: B
Response: Feelings of sudden, uncontrollable anxiety and the inability to breathe are classic symptoms of persons experiencing panic disorder.
Chapter: Anxiety Disorders

19. Martin is a 38-year-old patient with a long history of OCD, in which he must check that the door is locked for hours before leaving the house or going to bed at night. An appropriate nursing intervention for a patient with this disorder would be:
A. Restraining Martin in the recliner until he falls asleep
B. Requiring Martin to list the reasons why he must lock the doors repeatedly
C. Giving Martin a schedule to perform the this ritual
D. Offering Martin another behavior to substitute for this ritual
ANS: C
Response: People with OCD perform their ritual in order to relieve anxiety. They need to perform the specific behavior—and usually in a particular way. Behavior modification, which includes limiting the obsessive behavior and retraining the response to the anxiety, can be a positive nursing intervention for patients with OCD.
Chapter: Anxiety Disorders

20. Nurses know that patient needs that are not met will lead to anxiety. Anxiety leads to some sort of action by the patient. The action taken by the patient serves the purpose of:
A. Repression
B. Problem solving
C. Denial
D. Tension relief
ANS: D

Response: When tension is decreased, anxiety is decreased. Behaviors that reduce tension or anxiety are called primary gain behaviors.
Chapter: Anxiety Disorders

21. Your next door neighbor had a fire in his or her home last year. He accidentally left his coffeepot on and the cord caught on fire, causing a good amount of damage in his kitchen. Since then, he checks the coffeepot many times before leaving the house. "Sometimes I'm late for work," he laughs, as he tells you about the situation, "but I guess that's normal after having a fire, don't you think?" You know that this type of behavior is:
A. Normal. He has had a potentially life-threatening event.
B. Abnormal. He needs to "get over it." The fire was a long time ago.
C. Normal. He feels protective of his home.
D. Abnormal. This behavior is indicative of behaviors associated with OCD.
ANS: D
Response: He is showing signs of OCD. Even though the fire was a year ago and it is important to move on, the repetitive act is the mechanism that is reducing his stress at the moment.
Chapter: Anxiety Disorders

22. You are a home health nurse and are at a local pharmacy picking up a prescription for your client. As you leave the pharmacy, you observe a man forceably taking a woman's keys and her purse. She falls to the ground as he takes her car. You, of course, assist as much as you can, but you find yourself dreaming about the situation and are fearful to return to that pharmacy. You realize you may be exhibiting signs and symptoms of:
A. PTSD
B. Generalized anxiety disorder
C. Bipolar depression
D. Panic disorder
ANS: A
Response: These behaviors may be signs and symptoms of PTSD caused by witnessing the attack on the woman.
Chapter: Anxiety Disorders

Personality Disorders

1. Patients with antisocial personality disorder
A. Generally must have immediate gratification
B. Display a great deal of responsibility toward others
C. Display a great deal of anxiety
D. Have a great deal of self-control
ANS: A
Response: Individuals with antisocial personality disorder are generally self-centered and require immediate gratification of their needs.
Chapter: Personality Disorders

2. Individuals who have antisocial personality disorder do not usually have strong relationships or relate well with others because these patients have not learned to:
A. Trust
B. Communicate socially
C. Empathize with others
D. Accept praise
ANS: C
Response: Patients with antisocial personality disorder have an undeveloped or underdeveloped superego; therefore, they have not learned how to empathize (feel for someone else's situation) with others.
Chapter: Personality Disorders

3. A patient on the hospital's mental health floor has a diagnosis of borderline personality disorder. This patient is very convincing and talks another patient into sneaking out of the unit, "just to see if you can do it." When

confronted about the inappropriate nature of this behavior, the patient states, "Well someone was going to do it if I didn't!" A nurse recognizes this an as example of:
A. Transference
B. Denial
C. Repression
D. Rationalization
ANS: D
Response: Rationalization is one of the most commonly used defense mechanisms and is the most often used defense mechanism in people who have borderline personality disorders. A patient with borderline personality disorder shows no guilt.
Chapter: Personality Disorders

4. A patient who is diagnosed with passive-aggressive personality disorder has contracted with you to review the care plan. Your plan was to meet at 1330. At 1315 the patient informs you that this is not a convenient time and that 1430 would be much better for him or her. Your therapeutic response is:
A. Report the infraction to the physician
B. Inform the patient that contracts are to be kept and failure to do so will result in privileges being revoked
C. Compromise with the patient on a time
D. Send the patient back to the locked unit to think about his or her actions
ANS: B
Response: It is important for you to remain firm because this keeps the patient in reality and places the responsibility of his or her actions on the patient.
Chapter: Personality Disorders

5. Barbara is a new patient on your floor who is being assessed for several disorders, including suicide potential. You learn she attempts suicide every 6 to 12 months because she cannot tolerate living alone. She is unable to see two sides of a situation or an individual; they are either all good or all bad. You consider which of the following as a potential diagnosis for Barbara?
A. Borderline personality disorder
B. Multiple personality disorder
C. Narcissistic personality disorder
D. Antisocial personality disorder
ANS: A
Response: Patients with borderline personality disorders have difficulty accepting opposite qualities in the same situation and they have a strong fear of abandonment.
Chapter: Personality Disorders

6. A nice looking male patient is making suggestive comments to the female nursing staff. When he asks you for your phone number, you therapeutically respond:
A. "I do not believe in dating patients."
B. "It is against the rules for me to date patients."
C. "I'll think about it and let you know."
D. "You are very nice but our relationship is a professional one only."
ANS: D
Response: Your statement is accepting of the individual but it also assertively states a comfortable boundary between you and the patient.
Chapter: Personality Disorders

7. When planning care for an individual with borderline personality disorder, nurses realize that the patient
A. Will not be able to make decisions
B. Will expect special treatment
C. Will "act out" when feeling afraid or disrespected
D. Will withdraw and become uncommunicative
ANS: C
Response: The fear of abandonment is very strong in those with borderline personality disorders. Patients will demonstrate different inappropriate behaviors in order to call attention to their needs.
Chapter: Personality Disorders

8. A patient with borderline personality disorder approaches you and voices concern that he or she is being ignored and feels unimportant. The patient blames the nursing staff for these feelings because the nurses are "not paying attention" to him or her. Your best therapeutic response to this patient is:
A. "I will bring it up at our next meeting."
B. "It's all in your imagination."
C. "Tell me more about your feeling of 'being ignored.'"
D. "You need to share your feelings with the individual nurses you feel are ignoring you."
ANS: D
Response: By responding in this manner, you acknowledge the patient's concerns, but you also make the patient responsible for his or her actions. It is important for the nurse to avoid "getting in the middle" of these situations.
Chapter: Personality Disorders

9. The main mechanism used by patients who have personality disorders is:
A. Projection
B. Manipulation
C. Introjection
D. Repression
ANS: B
Response: Patients who have personality disorders display many defense mechanisms. The defense mechanism that seems to be present in all of the personality disorders is manipulation.
Chapter: Personality Disorders

10. Nurses understand that a major cause of personality disorders is:
A. Neurochemical imbalance
B. Genetics
C. Dysfunctional family relationships
D. Anoxia
ANS: C
Response: Dysfunctional families and ineffective maternal child bonding are the most frequently quoted reasons for the development of personality disorders in people.
Chapter: Personality Disorders

11. Nurses know that when working with patients who have personality disorders, the most difficult task for these patients will probably be:
A. Following rules
B. Getting along with others
C. Hoarding their medications
D. Participating in care plan meetings
ANS: B
Response: Developing and maintaining interpersonal relationships is a pervasive problem throughout personality disorders.
Chapter: Personality Disorders

12. A patient who is diagnosed with narcissistic personality disorder is constantly using the call light or following the nursing staff into other patient's rooms to ask, "Are you sure I look good? You know they can't get along without me at work. When can I leave here?" As the nurse caring for this patient, one of your goals for the patient will include all of the following *except*:
A. The patient will express reality about self-image.
B. The patient will require decreasing reinforcements from nursing staff.
C. The patient will acknowledge the feelings of others.
D. The patient will not be introspective about his or her condition.
ANS: D
Response: Patients with narcissistic personality disorders usually do not look within themselves. One goal of the nurse and patient is to have the patient learn to feel less threatened.

13. A patient's behavior is disruptive and causing many complaints from other patients. You approach this patient with which of the following techniques?
A. "Your behavior is not acceptable. You will need to remain in your room until you can behave more appropriately."
B. Ignore the behavior, since it is an uncontrollable part of the patient's illness
C. Set consistent limits on the patient's behavior
D. "You have a definite care plan. You must follow this plan; if you don't, you will be moved to a more structured unit."
ANS: C
Response: In order to avoid rejection from other patients on the unit, it is important to set limits on the patient's behavior. The patient needs to understand what is acceptable, what is unacceptable, and what the consequences are for inappropriate and disruptive behavior.
Chapter: Personality Disorders

14. People who have borderline personality disorders
A. Do not learn from past experiences and do not realize or care about the consequence of their behavior
B. Know the consequences of their behavior but do not care
C. Learn from past experiences and put that knowledge into practice.
D. Try to forget about past experiences
ANS: A
Response: People with borderline (sociopathic) personality disorders do not learn from past experiences, and either do not realize the consequences of their behavior on others or just do not care.
Chapter: Personality Disorders

15. Nancy has antisocial personality disorder. Which of the following is a goal of treatment for Nancy?
A. Comply with her medication regimen
B. Participate in long-term therapy
C. Become a group facilitator
D. Eliminate her anxiety
ANS: B
Response: People with antisocial personality disorders usually require long-term treatment.
Chapter: Personality Disorders

16. Tony is a 25-year-old male patient who is being treated at your hospital day-treatment center. Tony is very charming and seems popular. He has the ability to draw crowds around him, but you know he has been in trouble with the law several times since adolescence and lies constantly. You realize that Tony's behavior is reflective of:
A. Paranoid personality disorder
B. Schizoid personality disorder
C. Dependent personality disorder
D. Antisocial personality disorder
ANS: D
Response: People who have antisocial personality disorders have little respect for others and the law. They frequently have a record with the police.
Chapter: Personality Disorders

17. Cynthia is a patient who has been transferred to the mental health unit from the medical floor. She tells you that she "doesn't trust anyone" and she seems to be overly sensitive to constructive suggestions or comments made by staff and other patients. You suspect that her diagnosis will be:
A. Paranoid personality disorder
B. Antisocial personality disorder
C. Borderline personality disorder
D. Dependent personality disorder
ANS: A

Response: Cynthia's suspicion and mistrust are classic symptoms of paranoid personality disorder. People with this condition also tend to be emotionally hypersensitive.
Chapter: Personality Disorders

18. An appropriate nursing action/intervention for a patient with paranoid personality disorder is:
A. Give the patient advice on the correct decisions he or she should make.
B. Avoid giving clear answers about the patient's plan of care and treatment regimen.
C. Maintain clear and honest communication with the patient.
D. Restrict the number of social contacts for the patient.
ANS: C
Response: Patients with paranoid personality disorders have trouble trusting and believing in others. They need to trust that their nurses will be honest and consistent with them; they will learn to appreciate this.
Chapter: Personality Disorders

19. Janet is new to your medical unit. She is being treated for pelvic inflammatory disease, but she is uncooperative about answering your questions. You agree to let her settle in and you return in 30 minutes to find her very pleasant, agreeable, and almost docile. Over the course of the next 3 days, you witness these changes in Janet's personality. You also witness her "forgetting" to keep appointments and leaving lab specimens in unsecured areas. Not including her present medical condition, you begin to suspect that she may have which of the following personality disorders?
A. Antisocial/sociopathic
B. Passive-aggressive
C. Narcissistic
D. Dependent
ANS: B
Response: Janet is exhibiting some characteristics of passive-aggressive personality disorder. She is quiet and passive one moment and uncooperative the next. Patients with this condition will also "forget" to perform tasks asked of them and they may undermine other people or their medical treatment routine.
Chapter: Personality Disorders

20. Denise has been admitted to your medical unit for testing for migraines she has been having. She tells you about her several graduate degrees and points out to you that she really must be discharged soon, because her place of employment simply cannot function in her absence. Denise explains that she has won numerous awards, but that she "really didn't deserve them any more than anyone else who works with her." You request an evaluation from the mental health unit because your nursing assessment suggests a diagnosis of:
A. Dependent personality disorder
B. Schizoid personality disorder
C. Passive-aggressive personality disorder
D. Narcissistic personality disorder
ANS: D
Response: Denise is exhibiting characteristics of narcissistic personality disorder. She is recounting her personal attributes and attempting to make herself seem all-important, while at the same time expressing some form of unworthiness.
Chapter: Personality Disorders

21. You are caring for a patient in orthopedics who has a multiple fracture of the femur. The patient is also diagnosed with borderline personality disorder. Neither you nor any of the patient's family members are able to help the patient feel any pleasure. Inability to feel pleasure is called:
A. Hypomania
B. Anhedonia
C. Anoxia
D. Hedonism
ANS: B
Response: *Anhedonia* is the term for the inability to feel pleasure.
Chapter: Personality Disorders

22. Patients who seem shy, who seem to have few friends, and who may be described by others as "loners," may have which of the following personality disorders?
A. Dependent
B. Narcissistic
C. Schizoid
D. Paranoid
ANS: C
Response: People with schizoid personality disorders display all of these symptoms. It is important to remember, though, that not everyone who is shy or who has limited social contacts has a personality disorder.
Chapter: Personality Disorders

Schizophrenia

1. A patient in his mid-30s has a new diagnosis of schizophrenia and is taking chlorpromazine (Thorazine). Three days after beginning the chlorpromazine, he has jerky movements of his head and arms and he is concerned. The nurse assesses these symptoms as:
A. Extrapyramidal side effects
B. Dyspepsia
C. Torticollis
D. Dystonia
ANS: D
Response: "Dystonia" is an extrapyramidal side effect, but a more specific indicator of dystonia is the specific extrapyramidal side effect that the nurse will identify.
Chapter: Schizophrenia

2. "Hallucinations" are false sensory perceptions, which occur:
A. As a result of conflict
B. Without external stimulus
C. In schizophrenia only
D. Due to ineffective parenting
ANS: B
Response: Hallucinations are false sensory perceptions, which do not have external stimulus. Illusions occur as a result of perceptual stimulation.
Chapter: Schizophrenia

3. You notice a patient who seems to be listening to someone, but you do not see anyone else in the room. You interpret this behavior as a(n):
A. Illusion
B. Delusion
C. Hallucination
D. Confabulation
ANS: C
Response: The patient is experiencing a hallucination.
Chapter: Schizophrenia

4. Which of the following characteristics are most closely associated with schizophrenia?
A. Flat affect, autism, ambivalence, and loose associations
B. Bright affect, paranoia, and anhedonia
C. Autistic behavior and accuracy of perception
D. Insight, suspiciousness, and flight of ideas
ANS: A
Response: These characteristics are the "4 A's" of Eugene Bleuler, which are classic definitions of schizophrenia.
Chapter: Schizophrenia

5. A patient who is diagnosed with schizophrenia would display all of the following characteristics *except*:

A. Suspiciousness
B. Hallucinations
C. Flexibility of routine
D. Delusions
ANS: C
Response: Patients who are schizophrenic tend to be inflexible with their routines.
Chapter: Schizophrenia

6. A teenage patient is brought to your hospital by her parents. The patient exhibits unusual behaviors, including illogical thought processes and strange combinations of words that you do not understand. She is wearing dirty clothes and she has body odor. The patient also appears to carry on a conversation with a person who is not seen by you. Your first priority for this patient is:
A. Have her shower and change clothes
B. Bring her a snack
C. Resocialize her
D. Ensure her safety
ANS: D
Response: The patient's perception of reality may be impaired, because she is hallucinating. Safety is always the priority when a patient is not in touch with reality.
Chapter: Schizophrenia

7. Tim is a new patient to your mental health unit. He gets your attention, and when the two of you are alone he informs you that he "has the secret to eternal youth." He offers to tell you, but he is unable to because "they're out there hiding so they can steal it from me. I must be very careful." Your best therapeutic response to Tim is:
A. "Tim, I don't see anyone but you and me. It's time for dinner now. I'll walk with you to the dining room."
B. "Tim, nobody can have eternal youth. That's not realistic so don't talk about that anymore."
C. "I'd love to hear about it, Tim. Tell me your secret."
D. "I'll make sure 'they' are all gone, then you can tell me."
ANS: A
Response: You acknowledge Tim's statement, but honestly tell him there is nobody else there, while redirecting him to the here and now. This statement does not reinforce his delusion.
Chapter: Schizophrenia

8. Which of the following is the most appropriate nursing intervention for a patient with schizophrenia?
A. Teach the patient about the illness
B. Maintain consistency with the patient's plan of care
C. Insist that the patient participate in all activities provided on the unit
D. Allow the patient time to listen to the radio alone in his or her room
ANS: B
Response: Maintaining consistency in the patient's plan of care is the most important nursing intervention. The patient needs structure and consistent limits on for his or her behavior.
Chapter: Schizophrenia

9. A patient with a diagnosis of catatonic-type schizophrenia repeats words and phrases that someone else has just said. The nurse knows this repetitive speech pattern is:
A. Confabulation
B. Word salad
C. Echopraxia
D. Echolalia
ANS: D
Response: *Echolalia* is the term for this type of repetitive speech pattern. "Echopraxia" is repetition of another's motions.
Chapter: Schizophrenia

10. A patient has been admitted to the hospital. He or she has been telling the neighbors that someone is "bugging" the telephone line and listening in to all of his or her calls and thought processes. The patient is convinced that someone is "out to kill me" and is refusing to remove his or her clothing and wear the hospital gown during admission. As the nurse doing this admission, you:
A. Let the patient remain in his or her own clothing
B. Get the orderly to remove the patient's clothing
C. Get additional staff to help you remove the patient's clothing
D. Ask the patient why he or she is being so uncooperative
ANS: A
Response: It is important for the patient's psychological safety and for the rapport between you and the patient to allow him or her to wear his or her own clothing right now. You may try again later when the patient is calmer and more trusting. At this time, the patient will probably not be able to answer questions about his or her reasons for not removing the street clothing.
Chapter: Schizophrenia

11. Max says, "Nurse, see that man on the television? He is the reason why I am sick. He told them to make me this way." The nurse documents this as an episode of a(n):
A. Hallucination
B. Delusion
C. Illusion
D. Autistic thought
ANS: B
Response: Max's statement is an example of a delusion (a fixed, false belief).
Chapter: Schizophrenia

12. You have been floated to the surgical unit and are caring for a patient who has had a spinal fusion. The patient is receiving IV pain medication. You hear the patient calling out loudly about the "snakes crawling all over the bed." You consider several reasons for the patient's behavior, including drug reaction, electrolyte imbalance, and infection. In this case, your first priority is:
A. Call the doctor immediately
B. Report to the charge nurse immediately
C. Reassure the patient that there are no snakes and offer him or her a back rub
D. Stop the IV medication
ANS: A
Response: Because, in this case, the hallucination may be related to several etiologies, it is necessary to call the physician and continue to monitor and document any further symptoms.
Chapter: Schizophrenia

13. You observe a patient who has a diagnosis of schizophrenia. The patient is waiting for his or her significant other to arrive. When the visitor arrives, the patient tells the visitor that he or she is much too busy to talk right now, but at the same time the patient pulls another chair to the table. You note this as an example of:
A. Autism
B. Ambivalence
C. Appropriate affect
D. Anhedonia
ANS: B
Response: This is an example of conflicting needs occurring at the same time. The patient is trying to put distance in the relationship he or she has with the visitor while trying to bring the relationship between he or she and the visitor closer together.
Chapter: Schizophrenia

14. A patient who has schizophrenia suddenly verbally attacks you for being "one of them" and screams, "You are trying to hurt me, too!" Your most therapeutic response is:
A. "You know that is not true!"
B. Silence.
C. "I'd be angry, too. They are being terrible toward you!"
D. "It must be frightening to feel so threatened."

ANS: D

Response: This choice addresses the patient's need and states the patient's implied feeling. The statement allows the patient to begin discussion of the underlying problem and cause of the outburst.

Chapter: Schizophrenia

15. Mrs. R, the mother of a young schizophrenic patient, seeks you out and begins to cry. She expresses concern over her daughter's behavior. Your best response to this woman is:

A. "What is it that concerns you the most, Mrs. R."
B. "Well, you know, that is part of the illness."
C. "Here is a book on schizophrenia. This will help you."
D. "Are you afraid your daughter will always be like this?"

ANS: A

Response: This response narrows the focus of the mother's concern and allows you to immediately understand the main problem. Your response is also open-ended. Offering a book at this time is not the best choice, since the mother may not need it or may not be able to understand it. That kind of help can be used at a later time during the patient's hospitalization.

Chapter: Schizophrenia

16. When discharge teaching a patient who has schizophrenia and is taking clozapine (Clozaril), it is important to include all of the following *except*:

A. "Be sure to have you lab work on time and as ordered."
B. "Do not stop this drug abruptly. First call your doctor."
C. "Do not take any over-the-counter medications or alcohol while on this medication, without your doctor's approval."
D. "You may begin driving immediately, while taking this medication."

ANS: D

Response: This medication poses a risk of seizure activity; therefore, it is recommended to avoid driving or operating machinery while taking this medication.

Chapter: Schizophrenia

17. When discharging a schizophrenic patient who is taking haloperidol (Haldol), it is important for the nurse to advise the patient to:

A. Keep track of how much salt and water he or she consumes
B. Avoid exercise
C. Do not take any over-the-counter (OTC) medication without doctor approval.
D. Stop taking the medication if dry mouth develops and call the doctor immediately.

ANS: C

Response: Many OTC medications contain chemicals that can adversely interfere with the medicinal effect of haloperidol.

Chapter: Schizophrenia

18. Sally is experiencing an exacerbation of symptoms of her schizophrenia. She tells you, her nurse, that the voices are getting louder and that they are telling her to "walk in front of a big truck." Your first nursing action for Sally would be:

A. Divert her into a group activity immediately
B. Implement suicide precautions
C. Explain that there is nobody telling her to "walk in front of a big truck"
D. Notify her family and ask them if she has said this before

ANS: B

Response: Suicide precautions are called for as part of managing Sally's safety. She is hallucinating and is not in a state of reality. Safety is the nurse's first responsibility to the patient.

Chapter: Schizophrenia

19. You are one of the nurses monitoring the dining room during dinner. A male patient who has schizophrenia asks a table mate to "please pass the pepper." When the table mate does so, the first patient throws the pepper shaker at

you. He or she screams, "Now look what you've done! There are spiders all over my food! I can't eat this! Get the spiders out of there!" Your response is:
A. "Those aren't spiders; that is the pepper you asked for!"
B. "I don't see any spiders. Let's go to the game room for a little while before you try eating again."
C. "Where are the spiders? I am also afraid of them!"
D. "It is inappropriate to throw things; you need to go to the locked unit now."
ANS: B
Response: You have acknowledged the fact that you do not share the patient's perception, you have diverted the patient temporarily, and you have kept the patient in the reality that he or she will still need to eat dinner.
Chapter: Schizophrenia

20. Mrs. Jones has been taking chlorpromazine to combat the effects of her auditory hallucinations. Her response to you, which indicates that the medication is effective, is:
A. "There is more than one voice now!"
B. "They are whispering instead of talking loudly now!"
C. "I don't hear the voices now!"
D. "I only hear them sometimes, now."
ANS: C
Response: The medication is effective when the patient is free of the auditory hallucination.
Chapter: Schizophrenia

21. A new, yet unproven, theory relating to schizophrenia suggests that virues experienced by a woman during her pregnancy may contribute to the child's risk for having schizophrenia. You are preparing a young primipara who has read about this new theory. She asks you, "Nurse, how can I be sure my baby won't be crazy?" A helpful response to this young woman might be:
A. "We don't know the causes, so there's no way you can know."
B. "Crazy? Your baby won't be born 'crazy.'"
C. "Why are you so concerned?"
D. "The best defense for you right now is to take good care of yourself during your pregnancy. Please ask the doctor for more specific instructions on care."
ANS: D
Response: It is acceptable to encourage the woman to maintain good prenatal care, and it is legally appropriate to refer all specific questions to the physician.
Chapter: Schizophrenia

22. Which of the following is *not* a symptom of schizophrenia?
A. A flat or blunted affect
B. Neologisms (made-up words)
C. Autism
D. Effective and appropriate communication with others
ANS: D
Response: Communication is not effective and appropriate in most cases in patients with schizophrenia. All other responses provided *are* symptoms of schizophrenia.
Chapter: Schizophrenia

Organic Mental Disorders

1. Team members working with patients who have dementia need to have a common, unified approach because this type of patient requires:
A. Sameness and consistency in their lives
B. Strict rules and regulations
C. Behavior modification at all times
D. Staff who cannot be manipulated
ANS: A
Response: Consistency and relatively routine environments are important considerations to assist with reality orientation in persons who have dementia.
Chapter: Organic Mental Disorders

2. When preparing a care plan for a patient with a diagnosis of delirium, dementia, or cognitive impairment, the nurse will:
A. Increase mental and physical stimulus to improve mental function
B. State five current events from today's newspaper
C. Maintain consist daily routines
D. Encourage the patient to discuss memories from his or her childhood
ANS: C
Response: Consistency is important for reality orientation in cognitive disorders.
Chapter: Organic Mental Disorders

3. An elderly patient is admitted to your nursing home with a diagnosis of organic brain syndrome. This patient is frequently disoriented to person, place, and time. You expect to observe disorientation most frequently:
A. After a visit from the family
B. Upon awakening (in the morning, during the night, and so on)
C. During activities
D. On holidays
ANS: B
Response: Dimness of lighting, slowness to respond, and the experience of "sundowning" may all play a role in the frequency of disorientation upon awakening.
Chapter: Organic Mental Disorders

4. The best way to assist a patient who has mild Alzheimer's disease is:
A. Ask the physician to keep the patient sedated to avoid "acting out" behaviors
B. Provide strict one-on-one behavior modification techniques to prevent further cognitive deterioration
C. Encourage the family to begin preparations to move the person to a skilled nursing facility
D. Provide a stable, safe, and consistent environment
ANS: D
Response: Patients in the early stages of Alzheimer's disease are still quite functional, but providing consistency can maintain their safety and orientation during periods of forgetfulness or disorientation.
Chapter: Organic Mental Disorders

5. Nurses recognize that the main cause for Alzheimer's disease is:
A. Unknown at this time
B. Genetic
C. Related to use of aluminum cookware
D. Substance abuse
ANS: A
Response: Studies are being done, but there is no definitive cause for Alzheimer's disease.
Chapter: Organic Mental Disorders

6. A person who is receiving tests to confirm a diagnosis of Alzheimer's disease is preparing for a computerized tomography (CT) test. The patient becomes restless and is unable to follow the pre-examination directions given by the lab personnel. As the nurse who is assisting the patient, your best action at this time is:
A. Tell the patient that refusing to cooperate will require having to return another day
B. Give the patient the written instructions
C. Take the patient to a quiet waiting area until it is time for the CT scan
D. Make certain that the patient is tightly strapped to the examination table during the test
ANS: C
Response: Removing the patient from the activity and stimulation in the lab area will help lower the patient's anxiety and improve his or her ability to complete the examination.
Chapter: Organic Mental Disorders

7. You are the nurse caring for a patient with vascular-type dementia. When planning care for a person with this disorder, you should include:
A. Reeducation and behavior modification
B. Protective and supportive care
C. Resocialization and living skills training
D. Frequent participation in group activities
ANS: B
Response: Since brain cells do not regenerate, patients with vascular dementia will not greatly benefit from teaching or behavior modification. Only safety, comfort, and other supportive care are mandatory.
Chapter: Organic Mental Disorders

8. You are working with a patient who has dementia. The patient becomes withdrawn and negative. Your most therapeutic response to this patient is:
A. "Your family will feel very bad if you do not get along here!"
B. "Your doctor has ordered you to attend at least two activities each day."
C. "Would you prefer to stay alone in your room?"
D. "I need a partner to play cards with."
ANS: D
Response: Option "D" provides the most appropriate response because it simply and directly refocuses the patient to an activity without shaming, blaming, or threatening the patient. The patient also feels a sense of value to be sought out as a "partner."
Chapter: Organic Mental Disorders

9. A 65-year-old patient with vascular-type dementia is a high safety risk because he climbs out of bed, is unsteady on his feet, and frequently wanders. He is unable to remember instructions and has been found out of bed with the restraint tied around his neck. A team conference is called and you suggest:
A. "Let's ask the physician about the possibility of putting his mattress on the floor."
B. "Let's ask the physician for a stronger hypnotic."
C. "Let's ask the family what they would suggest."
D. "We could try four-point restraints at night."
ANS: A
Response: This suggestion is a safe and easy remedy that respects the patient's disorder and maintains some degree of independence for the patient.
Chapter: Organic Mental Disorders

10. George is a patient who has Alzheimer's disease. Three weeks after his admission, George's family asks you, "How long will it be before he is well again?" Your best response to them is:
A. "Soon. The doctor is trying new medications."
B. "There is no way to know that."
C. "What do you mean by 'better?'"
D. "He will continue to get progressively worse."
ANS: D
Response: This response is the best choice. While there is no way to predict a person's course, Alzheimer's disease is a progressive, degenerative illness and each person progresses through it differently.
Chapter: Organic Mental Disorders

11. Mavis Brown is a 75-year-old patient in your nursing home. She has Alzheimer's disease. Mavis comes to you at the desk one day and is crying. She says, "You all hate me. Everyone hates me!" Your therapeutic reply is:
A. "Nobody here hates you, Mavis."
B. "Why do you feel hated, Mavis?"
C. "You seem upset, Mavis. Let's go for a walk and talk."
D. "It's time for your medication, Mavis."
ANS: C
Response: You respond to the patient's feelings, show your concern, and redirect the patient's attention.
Chapter: Organic Mental Disorders

12. On of the main goals of the therapeutic milieu for the patient confused by delirium or dementia is:
A. Improve the patient's interpersonal skills
B. Help the patient to feel "at home"
C. Help the staff to help the patient
D. Help the patient to see others' problems
ANS: A
Response: One goal of the therapeutic environment is to help the patient improve interpersonal skills and the way he or she relates to other people.
Chapter: Organic Mental Disorders

13. Henry Smith is 88-years-old and has been having periods of disorientation and confusion that worsen at night. He has been given a diagnosis of Alzheimer's disease. When you pick up Henry's tray after supper, you observe that he has not touched any of the food. As his nurse, you understand that:
A. He is too depressed to eat
B. He sees ants in his food
C. He is too forgetful to remember to eat
D. He is deliberately obstinate
ANS: C
Response: Henry's short-term memory is affected. He needs reminders, cues, and supervision to help him remember to eat.
Chapter: Organic Mental Disorders

14. Nurses who work with patients who have cognitive disorders know that the current trend in treatment is to:
A. Maintain the patients in their community as long as possible
B. Medicate the patients with high doses of antianxiety medications
C. Provide the patients with intensive occupational therapy
D. Make the patients responsible for their own actions and decisions
ANS: A
Response: The current trend is to keep patients in their community as long as possible. Patients, family members, and the medical staff should work together toward this patient outcome.
Chapter: Organic Mental Disorders

15. Nurses understand that patients with dementia demonstrate all of the following *except*:
A. A lack of concentration
B. A resistance to change
C. An attention to personal care and appearance
D. A preference to dwell in the past
ANS: C
Response: Patients with dementia seldom take interest in their appearance or hygiene.
Chapter: Organic Mental Disorders

16. Which of the following activities would be most appropriate for a patient who is in the moderate stage of Alzheimer's disease?
A. A large jigsaw puzzle
B. Trivial Pursuit
C. A scavenger hunt
D. Playing a game of catch with a soft ball
ANS: D
Response: Playing catch is not cognitively demanding, but it does provide exercise and tactile stimulation.
Chapter: Organic Mental Disorders

17. When planning interventions for a patient who has Alzheimer's disease, the nurse knows that patients with this disorder

A. Will remember teaching that was done yesterday

B. Will most likely have moderate to severe memory impairment

C. Will perform required tasks (such as dressing, grooming, and so on)

D. Will respond well to rigid schedules

ANS: B

Response: Instructions should be short and concise. The nurse should not expect the patient, even with the best of instruction, to remember the instruction or carry out the required task.

Chapter: Organic Mental Disorders

18. "Sundowner's syndrome" or "sundowning" is a condition frequently seen in patients with organic mental disorders. *Sundowning* can best be described as:

A. Compulsion to watch the sun set

B. Sleeping 12 hours per day

C. Reversing day and night behavior (sleeping during the day and staying awake during the night)

D. Staying awake for several days at a time

ANS: C

Response: "Sundowner's syndrome" or "sundowning" is a condition of having traditional day and night behavior reversed. Patients with Sundowner's syndrome typically sleep during the day hours and are awake during the night hours.

Chapter: Organic Mental Disorders

19. The best nursing action when caring for an elderly patient who exhibits sundowner's syndrome is:

A. Ask the doctor to increase the patient's sleeping medication at bedtime

B. Ask the patient why he or she does not sleep at night

C. Wake the patient when you see him or her sleeping during the day

D. Keep the lights on in the patient's room at night

ANS: D

Response: Keeping the light on will promote the patient's safety upon awakening at night. Interrupting daytime naps is more effective for a young person than it is for an older person.

Chapter: Organic Mental Disorders

20. One of the symptoms seen in patients who have Alzheimer's disease is confabulation. *Confabulation* is best described as:

A. Forgetfulness

B. Low self-esteem

C. Making up a story to fill gaps in memory

D. Teasing behavior

ANS: C

Response: Patients who confabulate are realizing that there are lapses in their memory. They make up plausible stories to fill in these gaps in memory, in an effort to "hide" them.

Chapter: Organic Mental Disorders

21. Your Alzheimer's unit is planning to update its surroundings. All staff, family, and patients have input at the planning meetings. Some tenets that remain constant for providing safe and appropriate care for patients with Alzheimer's-type dementia are:

A. Medications often have side effects that may be counter-productive to treatment.

B. There is no substitute for appropriate programming.

C. Colorful changes in certain areas, such as carpeting in the hallways, may actually confuse patients and may lead to falls or fear to physically move past that change of color.

D. All of the above

ANS: D

Response: All of these statements are true.

Chapter: Organic Mental Disorders

22. A family member asks about using an experimental treatment on her loved one who is a resident in your facility. The relative is specifically interested in new studies relating estrogen use to decreased symptoms of Alzheimer's disease. The team members may respond to the family member appropriately by saying:
A. "Yes, studies are being done but to date, there is no proof that estrogen decreases the symptoms of Alzheimer's disease. Please talk with the patient's doctor."
B. "Yes, it looks like they have found the cure for Alzheimer's disease through the use of estrogen."
C. "Yes, we, as a unit, are suggesting that all patients and their families ask their doctors to prescribe estrogen."
D. None of the above
ANS: A
Response: To date, there is absolutely no conclusive evidence that estrogen therapy is effective in either preventing Alzheimer's disease or decreasing the symptoms associated with it. Patients and families should seek the advice of their physician.
Chapter: Organic Mental Disorders

Somatoform Disorders

1. Mr. Stiff has a paralysis of his right leg for which his doctor cannot find a physiologic cause. You suspect that the patient will be diagnosed with a(n):
A. Conversion disorder
B. Hypochondriac disorder
C. Somatization disorder
D. Malingering
ANS: A
Response: Paralysis and loss of sight, for which there are no physical causes, are classic symptoms of "conversion disorder."
Chapter: Somatoform Disorders

2. Nurses realize that in conversion disorder, the patient:
A. Lets go of emotionally uncomfortable thoughts and feelings
B. Expresses thoughts and feelings through physical symptoms
C. Understands the cause for the paralysis
D. Projects the problem onto a significant other
ANS: B
Response: The patient is eliminating the underlying anxiety by expressing it in physical terms. This is a form of "primary gain."
Chapter: Somatoform Disorders

3. You are preparing a care plan for a patient who is experiencing blindness as a symptom of conversion disorder. You know:
A. It is appropriate to ignore the patient's concerns about the blindness
B. The patient is intentionally producing the symptoms, so you institute behavior guidelines
C. The patient is exhibiting manifestations of a psychological problem
D. This is a sign of a personality flaw
ANS: C
Response: The patient is not able to control the symptoms, which are expressions of the patient's emotional pain.
Chapter: Somatoform Disorders

4. A young adult patient is admitted for further testing and treatment of bilateral leg paralysis. The preliminary diagnosis is conversion disorder. A nurse's knowledge of this disorder indicates that the patient will most likely:
A. Recover use of his or her legs while in the hospital, but experience a return of paralysis when under stress again
B. Recover use of his or her legs without the threat of reoccurrence
C. Experience the paralysis "traveling" to other limbs
D. Express understanding of the paralysis in relation to his or her stress
ANS: A
Response: The patient will most likely "recover" from the paralysis when the emotional threat is removed but may experience it again when a stressful situation arises in the future.
Chapter: Somatoform Disorders

5. A 30-year-old patient is admitted to the medical floor with paralysis of both legs, etiology unknown. The patient is given a diagnosis of "conversion disorder." As a nurse caring for this patient, you would expect this patient to be:
A. Extremely depressed
B. Calm and lucid
C. Concerned about the sudden paralysis
D. Nervous and unable to sit quietly
ANS: B
Response: People who have conversion disorder quite literally "convert" their anxiety into the symptom. When the symptom develops, it "replaces" the anxiety and acts as a defense against the anxiety. The patient has no "need" to feel the anxiety.
Chapter: Somatoform Disorders

6. Nurses understand the symptoms of conversion disorder, such as blindness or paralysis, act as:
A. Attention-getting mechanisms
B. Diversions
C. Signals to learn to focus on other things
D. Mechanisms to deal with severe conflict or anxiety
ANS: D
Response: Anxiety is unconsciously converted into these severe symptoms in an effort to avoid confronting the anxiety.
Chapter: Somatoform Disorders

7. Mr. M has been admitted to the medical unit with a diagnosis of "peptic ulcer." Nurses understand that peptic ulcers may be considered a somatoform disorder because peptic ulcers are:
A. Physical illnesses caused by an underdeveloped psyche
B. Emotionally based disorders of unknown cause
C. Physical disorders strongly related to long-term emotional stress
D. Psychological disorders caused by fear
ANS: C
Response: There is a strong correlation between the existence of stress over a long period of time and the development, or at least the predisposition, for development of peptic ulcers. There are also other causal factors in the development of peptic ulcers.
Chapter: Somatoform Disorders

8. Patient W has been a patient on your medical unit for 4 days. Patient W's main symptoms included sudden blindness and paralysis of all fingers. Medical diagnosis has been negative; patient W has been given the diagnosis of "conversion disorder." (An) appropriate nursing action(s) for patient W would be:
A. Let patient W know that you understand the symptoms are real to him or her
B. Discuss the physical symptoms with patient W in detail
C. Understand that there is no need to report or record new physical "complaints" because you now know the condition is not "medical" in nature
D. Reinforce the secondary gain, because you know doing so is beneficial to the patient's recovery
ANS: A
Response: It is important for the patient to feel that the nurse understands that the symptoms are real to him or her and it is appropriate to redirect the patient's attention to other activities or topics. It is not appropriate, however, to focus on the patient's symptoms. Any change of condition is always important to record and report (for any patient or any condition).
Chapter: Somatoform Disorders

9. The somatoform condition in which symptoms include pain that changes location frequently, depression, and most often present before or approximately at age 30 is:
A. Hypochondriasis
B. Somatization disorder

C. Body dysmorphic disorder
D. Conversion disorder
ANS: B
Response: The symptoms are characteristic of somatization disorder.
Chapter: Somatoform Disorders

Substance-Related Disorders

1. Mr. Thomas, who is 50-years-old, is being treated for pneumonia and dehydration. He has a history of alcoholism and admits to starting to drink heavily again. He tells you, "I'm a horrible person. My family deserves someone better than me to care for them." Your most therapeutic response to him is:
A. "It sounds as though you are feeling guilty about drinking, Mr. Thomas."
B. "What makes you say that you are a horrible person, Mr. Thomas?"
C. "I'm sure that your family is satisfied, Mr. Thomas."
D. "Well, you're here now and you quit drinking once. You will quit again if you want to."
ANS: A
Response: The nurse "parrots" or "reflects" the patient's own words to encourage him to discuss his feelings. He has already stated what makes him feel "horrible."
Chapter: Substance-Related Disorders

2. You are caring for a patient who has a long history of alcohol abuse. Recently, this patient went on a 5-day drinking binge, of which he or she has no memory. This is an example of:
A. Selective memory
B. Wernicke's syndrome
C. Blackout
D. Denial
ANS: C
Response: The patient admitting to amnesia for the events that occurred during the period of heavy alcohol use. This amnesia is called "blackout."
Chapter: Substance-Related Disorders

3. Nurses understand that in people who are addicted to alcohol, the person who is most responsible for the patient's recovery is the
A. Psychiatrist
B. Nurse
C. Group leader
D. Patient
ANS: D
Response: The patient who is addicted to alcohol or other substances is ultimately responsible for his or her recovery.
Chapter: Substance-Related Disorders

4. You are socializing with a group of nurses that you work with on a routine basis. Terri is getting very loud and tells you that she usually has six or eight beers most evenings. She is defensive about your reaction to the amount of alcohol she consumes. She says, "I have days where I can't remember what happened the night before, sure, but only once in a while." If you were a nurse caring for Terri, the best action you could suggest to her is:
A. "Maybe you should stop at four beers, Terri."
B. "Have a friend make you stop at four beers, Terri."
C. "Terri, you have been diagnosed as an alcoholic. You would benefit by using no alcohol at all."
D. "Terri, have you considered 'near-beer'?"
ANS: C
Response: You are honest and state the facts to Terri. The other options either remove the responsibility from the patient or provide a "substitute" for the alcohol, which is often contraindicated in treatment.
Chapter: Substance-Related Disorders

5. You assess a patient for delirium tremens (DTs) and look for which of the following sets of symptoms?
A. Confusion, hallucination, agitation, and fine tremors
B. Denial, manipulation, and combativeness
C. Depression, remorse, and withdrawal from reality
D. Suspicion, mania, and stubbornness
ANS: A
Response: These are the key symptoms of DTs.
Chapter: Substance-Related Disorders

6. You are caring for a young patient who has been shot and has had surgery to remove the bullet fragments. The patient is not responding to the pain medications ordered by the doctor and admits to being addicted to street drugs. The doctor changes the patient's medication to methadone, which:
A. Eliminates the addiction to the street drugs
B. Can be legally dispensed and controlled
C. Maintains pain control without causing addiction
D. Is especially effective for gunshot wounds
ANS: B
Response: Methadone is a legal drug that can be legally prescribed and dispensed. Strict records are kept, as with all narcotics use. The drug is used to help addicts recover but is not without it's own potential for addiction.
Chapter: Substance-Related Disorders

7. "Hard" drugs, such as cocaine, cause dependence easily because they
A. Are analgesics
B. Clear thinking processes
C. Decrease motor activity
D. Blunt reality
ANS: D
Response: The "hard" drugs help the user to avoid true feelings and perceptions of reality. These drugs provide a chemical escape, which the user becomes dependent on.
Chapter: Substance-Related Disorders

8. Randi is a young model. She had been taking high doses of amphetamines to keep her weight down for her profession, but she is now experiencing amphetamine withdrawal. She presented to the clinic with which of the following sets of symptoms of amphetamine withdrawal?
A. Chest pain, palpitations, and diaphoresis
B. Depression, rhinorrhea, and sluggishness
C. Euphoria, hyperactivity, and hyperalertness
D. Diaphoresis, clammy palms, and diarrhea
ANS: B
Response: Depressive symptoms and a "runny nose" that is similar to an allergic reaction are classic symptoms of amphetamine withdrawal.
Chapter: Substance-Related Disorders

9. A young adult arrives in the after-hours clinic with euphoria, dilated pupils, an elevated heart rate, and fine tremors of the hands. The patient admits to recent use of an illegal street drug. As the nurse collecting this data, you suspect:
A. LSD
B. "Crack" cocaine
C. Amphetamines
D. Downers
ANS: C
Response: The patient's symptoms are consistent with the increase in motor and psychic response that occurs with amphetamine use.
Chapter: Substance-Related Disorders

10. Nurses expect the basic personality quality of a person who is addicted to drugs or alcohol to be:
A. Underactive id and strong self-esteem
B. Overactive ego and the ability to delay gratification
C. Underactive id and the ability to delay gratification
D. Low self-esteem and the inability to delay gratification
ANS: D
Response: People who become dependent on substances tend to have low self-esteem and need immediate gratification. They also tend to fear stressful situations.
Chapter: Substance-Related Disorders

11. Nurses working with patients who are alcoholic are aware that which of the following classifications of medication is generally contraindicated
A. Antianxiety medications
B. Nonsteroidal anti-inflammatory medications
C. Antidepressant medications
D. Antipsychotic medications
ANS: A
Response: Antianxiety medications ("minor tranquilizers") have a high potential for physical and psychological dependence and are contraindicated in patients who are dependent on alcohol or chemical substances.
Chapter: Substance-Related Disorders

12. Alcohol is a(n):
A. Central nervous system (CNS) stimulant
B. CNS depressant
C. Antipsychotic
D. Antidepressant
ANS: B
Response: Alcohol is a CNS depressant. It may initially give the illusion of being a stimulant, but it will eventually slow body systems and, if used to extremes or in conjunction with other sedative medications, may cause death.
Chapter: Substance-Related Disorders

13. You are caring for a female patient who is a long-term alcoholic. She screams, "Get the bugs off of my skin. I feel them all over my body! Get them off!" She is experiencing what type of hallucination?
A. Auditory
B. Visual
C. Taste
D. Tactile
ANS: D
Response: Feeling "bugs" or other objects on the skin is an example of a tactile hallucination. Any of the five senses can be affected when a patient hallucinates.
Chapter: Substance-Related Disorders

14. A 35-year-old male patient signs in as a voluntary commitment for treatment for drug abuse. He strongly maintains that he does not have a problem and states, "I'm only here because my boss threatened to fire me if I didn't come in." The *best* nursing response to this patient is:
A. "I wonder why your boss said that, if you don't have a problem?"
B. "From your perspective, what do you think is the most important information for me to know about you?"
C. "Your boss sounds pretty harsh!"
D. "Well, you are here on your own, so you can leave whenever you want to."
ANS: B
Response: This is the nurse's best response because it allows the patient to set the direction of the conversation. This response also gives the nurse an idea of the patient's priority for treatment.
Chapter: Substance-Related Disorders

15. A patient has completed treatment for alcoholism. If treatment was successful, a nurse might expect which of the following outcome statements from this patient upon discharge?
A. "Now, if my family will just be good, I won't be back!"
B. "I just know I can have an occasional drink and be fine. I know how to handle it now."
C. "I realize that Alcoholics Anonymous will always be a requirement. I am responsible for my own sobriety."
D. "I am so glad I found out what my problem is. I am cured now!"
ANS: C
Response: Patients who are addicted to alcohol require continuous support in the form of a group such as Alcoholics Anonymous. Recovery is a process, not an absolute event at the end of a treatment regimen.
Chapter: Substance-Related Disorders

16. *Drug abuse* can be defined as:
A. Excessive use of a drug that is not consistent with usual medical practice
B. A physical dependence
C. A psychological dependence
D. A compulsion to take the drug
ANS: A
Response: Drug abuse is the act of excessive use or misuse of a drug that is not consistent with standard medical applications for that drug.
Chapter: Substance-Related Disorders

17. Nurses are aware that people who abuse alcohol and drugs
A. Are of low-socioeconomic groups
B. Use only the drug of their choice
C. Use more than one drug and are often also alcoholic
D. Are all alcoholics before they begin using other drugs
ANS: C
Response: Frequently, people who are addicted to drugs are addicted to more than one drug and are also abusers of alcohol.
Chapter: Substance-Related Disorders

18. A patient is brought to the hospital while withdrawing from alcohol intoxication and abuse of diazepam (Valium). Your *first* nursing intervention for this patient is:
A. Immediate participation in an Alcoholics Anonymous meeting
B. Lockup until the symptoms of withdrawal have subsided
C. Have the patient verbalize feelings about what led to the chemical abuse
D. Monitoring of vital signs and providing safety and emotional support
ANS: D
Response: This patient is under the influence of two drugs, which are CNS depressants and may potentiate each other. Physical and medical safety and stabilization are required for this patient. Emotional support and acceptance are also required. Verbalization of feelings will be important later, but not as a primary intervention in this instance.
Chapter: Substance-Related Disorders

19. A patient comes to the clinic asking for help and admits to trying cocaine "just once, but I got hooked!" This patient is here now because "I just watched a friend die! I don't want to do that. You've got to help me!" You know that people who withdraw from cocaine will have cravings for the drug. They will also experience:
A. Depression
B. Mania
C. Paranoia
D. Dilated pupils
ANS: A
Response: People who are in withdrawal from cocaine will experience depression that can last a year.
Chapter: Substance-Related Disorders

20. A co-worker is a heavy user of alcohol. This co-worker announces, "Do I ever have a hangover today!" You are concerned about the amount of alcohol consumption and you expect which of the following symptoms of hangover?
A. Giddiness and euphoria
B. Hypoglycemia
C. Blood alcohol level of 2.0 or higher
D. Headache, gastritis, and irritability
ANS: D
Response: The symptoms of hangover are generally unpleasant and include headache, gastrointestinal implications, fatigue, and irritability.
Chapter: Substance-Related Disorders

21. Tori, a 16-year-old student, is accompanied to the school health service by a counselor. She has been disruptive in class and the teacher thinks Tori has been using marijuana. Tori laughs at the teacher and says, "Man, it's just some spices." You have just read some new information and consider Tori might be using:
A. "Bidi" or "rokok," which is a type of spiced and flavored cigarettes
B. PCP
C. Alcohol
D. All of the above
ANS: D
Response: There is not enough information to positively identify or rule out use of any of the stated substances.
Chapter: Substance-Related Disorders

22. Factors associated with the popularity of "bidi" or "rokok" among adolescents include pleasant taste, low cost, and
A. Increased amounts of carbon monoxide
B. Decreased inhaling
C. Lower amounts of tar and nicotine
D. All of the above
ANS: A
Response: These hand-rolled cigarettes are high in carbon monoxide. They have a higher percentage of tar and nicotine than conventional cigarettes (estimates are as high as three times the amount compared to conventional cigarettes).
Chapter: Substance-Related Disorders

Eating Disorders

1. Nurses working with patients who have eating disorders should:
A. Encourage patients to identify the thoughts and feelings underlying the disorder
B. Do a strict intake, output, and calorie count for each shift
C. Keep patients in view for 1 to 2 hours after meals
D. Have a staff person monitoring each table during meals
ANS: A
Response: The underlying thoughts and feelings of these patients led to the disorder and are important to explore. Nurses should not strictly focus on the food.
Chapter: Eating Disorders

2. Your first goal in the care of a patient with an eating disorder is:
A. Reassure the patient that his or her body is very well built
B. Teach the patient nutrition requirements for his or her age and height
C. Establish a trusting relationship with the patient
D. Ask the patient to explain why he or she will not eat
ANS: C
Response: It is imperative to develop a trusting nurse-patient relationship in order to get the cooperation of the patient.
Chapter: Eating Disorders

3. You are getting data from a 15-year-old girl who has been brought to the clinic by her mother. The girl has an eating disorder and has lost 15 lb in 8 days. The patient looks at you and states, "You are the only one who tries to understand!" Your response to her would be:
A. "I'm sure your mother understands."
B. "What is that you want people to understand?"
C. "Have you tried to talk to your family?"
D. "Why do you think I understand you?"
ANS: B
Response: You attempt to get the patient to clarify her concerns without giving her an opportunity to use other defense mechanisms or minimizing her feelings.
Chapter: Eating Disorders

4. Nurses understand that the underlying belief of patients who have "anorexia" is that being thin will:
A. Decrease their problems
B. Make them smarter
C. Increase their control over other people
D. Increase their popularity and acceptance
ANS: D
Response: Patients with eating disorders equate "thin" with "pretty" and "popular." This is important to them. The control issue is control over self, not others.
Chapter: Eating Disorders

5. An appropriate goal for a patient who is on behavior modification for anorexia nervosa is:
A. Gain 1 lb per week
B. Eat all food at each meal
C. Discuss the meaning of food to the patient for 1 hour every day
D. Attend therapeutic cooking classes daily
ANS: A
Response: Patients with anorexia nervosa need to gain weight. Setting a specific weight-gain goal is appropriate for behavior modification programs.
Chapter: Eating Disorders

6. Mark is a male model who has been admitted for weight loss and dehydration. Mark tells you, "I can eat anything I want and I don't gain weight. Isn't that great?" After dinner you hear a noise and you observe Mark vomiting in the bathroom. You document this and suspect:
A. Food poisoning
B. Anorexia nervosa
C. Bulimia nervosa
D. Paranoia about the meal
ANS: C
Response: Vomiting and preoccupation with appearance are the two main symptoms of "bulimia nervosa."
Chapter: Eating Disorders

7. You notice that a patient you are caring for who has been in the hospital for 3 weeks for treatment of bulimia nervosa continues to purge (vomit) when feeling stressed. Your best action to help would be:
A. Stay with the patient after meals as a gentle reminder not to purge
B. Tell the patient you will report him/her to the psychiatrist for failure to work with his or her program
C. Excuse the patient from one therapy session daily for 1 week to decrease stress
D. Remind the patient you are there to help, but he or she has to take responsibility for his or her progress
ANS: D
Response: It is the patient's responsibility to get well; nurses and therapists are only tools in the healing process. Significant behaviors do need to be reported and documented, but the patient must be reminded about self-responsibility.
Chapter: Eating Disorders

8. You are part of a team who cares for patients with eating disorders. As a team, what is the main priority in the care plan for someone with an eating disorder?
A. Meeting on a daily basis to discuss manipulative behaviors you observe in the patient
B. Restrict the patient to bedrest until the first weight-gain goal is reached
C. Allow unlimited exercise and weight training
D. Weigh the patient twice daily
ANS: A
Response: Patients with eating disorders can be extremely manipulative and it is important that the health care team routinely communicates about behaviors that the patient could be using that are counterproductive to treatment.
Chapter: Eating Disorders

9. You have a 14-year-old son who plays with his food at mealtime. He seldom eats and when he does, he only eats tiny bites. This has been going on for 2 months. As a nurse and a parent, you begin to suspect anorexia nervosa and you know that your son
A. Eats large amounts of food several times daily
B. Can enjoy food; he's just in a stage right now
C. Fears being fat
D. Is constantly hungry
ANS: C
Response: People who have anorexia are extremely afraid of being fat. They generally have an aversion to food and are not hungry, or will deny feeling hungry.
Chapter: Eating Disorders

10. Nurses know that the main difference between "anorexia nervosa" and "bulimia nervosa" is that the patient with bulimia nervosa:
A. Is obese and is trying to lose excess weight
B. Realizes that he or she has a problem and is trying to hide it
C. Has a distorted body image and does not see himself or herself as others see him or her
D. Has had ineffective parenting
ANS: B
Response: Patients who have bulimia nervosa realize they have a problem, but try to hide it and correct it themselves; however, they know they are out of control and unable to correct the condition.
Chapter: Eating Disorders

11. A 14-year-old patient is diagnosed with anorexia nervosa. Nurses know the cause of this disorder is usually:
A. Poor parenting
B. Anger at parents
C. Low self-esteem
D. Distorted body image
ANS: D
Response: The cause for "anorexia nervosa" is a distorted appearance, rather than low self-esteem. The patient feels and perceives him or herself as "fat" no matter what the actual body weight.
Chapter: Eating Disorders

12. Rob, a 15-year-old, has lost 30 lb in 3 months. Rob is 6 ft tall and weighs 110 lb. He is aspiring to be a model and he tells you that he is "fat. Just look at how puffy my feet and arms still are. I have to get rid of the fat there."
The priority nursing diagnosis you choose for Rob is:
A. Body image disturbance: distorted perception
B. Knowledge deficit: nutritional requirements
C. Altered nutrition, more than body requirements
D. Potential for suicide
ANS: A
Response: Patients with anorexia nervosa have an altered body image. There is no indication at this point that this patient is suicidal.
Chapter: Eating Disorders

13. Which nursing diagnosis is *best* for a patient with bulimia nervosa?
A. Knowledge deficit related to body weight
B. Denial of condition related to need for acceptance by peers
C. Cognitive impairment related to illness
D. Fluid imbalance: more than body requirements
ANS: B
Response: The need to be accepted by the peer group can lead to denial of the severity of bulimia nervosa.
Chapter: Eating Disorders

14. The main difference between "anorexia nervosa" and "bulimia nervosa" is that in bulimia nervosa, the patient is:
A. Obese and seriously attempting to lose weight
B. Grossly underweight but still sees his or her body as being fat
C. Aware that he or she has a problem but is not able to control it
D. Rebelling against his or her parents
ANS: C
Response: Patients who have bulimia nervosa know they have a problem and are unable to control it. The behaviors of hiding their eating habits and the binge-purge cycle are indicators of the patient's realization that this is unhealthy behavior.
Chapter: Eating Disorders

15. Nurses realize the importance of family relationships in the life of a patient with anorexia nervosa. As a nurse, you would expect which of the following attitudes or behaviors in the parents of an adolescent with anorexia nervosa?
A. Indifferent and inattentive
B. Permissive and providing loose boundaries
C. Immature and concerned with themselves
D. Overly protective and rigid
ANS: D
Response: Parents with children who develop anorexia nervosa tend to have personalities and parenting styles that are rigid, unyielding, and overly protective.
Chapter: Eating Disorders

16. When preparing a therapeutic milieu for a patient who has bulimia nervosa the nurse should provide:
A. Realistic limits and guidelines
B. A controlling atmosphere
C. Constant focus on the correct type and amount of food
D. Sympathy for the patient's condition
ANS: A
Response: The treatment milieu for a patient who has bulimia nervosa must set boundaries and guidelines, which are consistent and reasonable. These boundaries and guidelines decrease anxiety and increase the patient's trust and willingness to participate in treatment.
Chapter: Eating Disorders

17. You are the nurse caring for a 20-year-old female patient who is being treated for bulimia nervosa. You realize that the activity of bingeing and purging for several months has placed this patient at a high risk for:
A. Bowel obstruction
B. Cardiac arrhythmias and electrolyte imbalances
C. Asthma and food allergies
D. Throat cancer
ANS: B
Response: Purging at such a high frequency, as when a person is suffering from bulimia nervosa, puts the patient at risk for electrolyte imbalances and the cardiac complications (which arise from the electrolyte imbalances).
Chapter: Eating Disorders

18. A 15-year-old female is 15 lb underweight. She believes she is grossly overweight and she exercises vigorously 5 to 6 hours a day. She is a straight-A student in school and is the lead singer in her school choir and musical theater group. She is well liked by adults, but she has few friends of her own age group. Your nursing assessment of this patient leads you to the potential nursing diagnosis of:
A. Conversion disorder
B. Paranoid schizophrenia
C. Generalized anxiety disorder
D. Eating disorder
ANS: D
Response: This patient is exhibiting many of the classic symptoms of one of the eating disorders.
Chapter: Eating Disorders

19. In addition to gastrointestinal disorders associated with eating disorders, nurses must be aware of and assess for other medical complications including:
A. Electrolyte imbalances
B. Cardiac irregularities
C. Dehydration
D. All of the above
ANS: D
Response: All of the listed choices are potential medical complications for eating disorders that nurses should be constantly aware of. Electrolyte imbalances can also be a cause of unusual behavior.
Chapter: Eating Disorders

Suicide

1. A patient becomes suicidal and is transferred to the locked unit of your hospital. Because this patient is suicidal you should:
A. Keep the patient in your line of vision at all times
B. Perform suicide assessments every half-hour
C. Inform the doctor that the patient is now in a locked area
D. Take vital signs every 15 minutes
ANS: A
Response: Patients who are suicidal should be under constant supervision. It is important to stay in close physical proximity to the patient who is suicidal.
Chapter: Suicide

2. Patients are most likely to commit suicide when:
A. They are severely depressed.
B. The depression is lifting
C. They are recently discharged from the hospital
D. They have a significant other who is supportive
ANS: B
Response: When depression begins to lift, the patient has more energy and is better able to plan and carry out the act of suicide.
Chapter: Suicide

3. As you perform a suicide assessment on your patient, you learn that the patient has only one person to call in times of need, has been thinking about suicide frequently in past weeks, and has attempted suicide once before. You believe this patient's suicide risk is:
A. Low
B. Moderate
C. Guarded
D. Imminent
ANS: B
Response: The patient does not have a definite plan, but the fact that suicide has been tried at least once before puts this patient at moderate risk for attempting suicide.

4. The best approach a nurse can use to gain information relating to a patient's potential for suicide is:
A. "What do you plan to be doing five years from now?"
B. "Does your family know you are considering suicide?"
C. "What have other patients told you about their suicide attempts?"
D. "I would like to know if you are thinking of killing yourself now."
ANS: D
Response: Option "D" asks for the patient to discuss his or her thoughts about suicide and deals only with the patient's immediate concern. The patient may not be able to discuss the future while in a state of crisis.
Chapter: Suicide

5. When planning care for a patient who is suicidal, the nurse knows:
A. Suicide attempts are only gestures.
B. Suicide is a crime and must be reported to the authorities.
C. Teaching new problem-solving skills is a priority of care for suicidal patients.
D. It is necessary to know the reasons why the patient has suicidal thoughts.
ANS: C
Response: Patients who are suicidal have lost the ability to see potential options. Teaching systems for problem solving is a way to help the patient help him or herself.
Chapter: Suicide

6. It is necessary to place one of your patients on suicide precautions. The most therapeutic way to implement these precautions is:
A. One-on-one care of that patient
B. Keep the patient in his or her room at all times
C. Make an obvious attempt at removing all potentially dangerous objects from the treatment milieu
D. Tell the patient he or she has one more chance to verbalize his or her feelings about the current situation or will be transferred to the lock-up unit
ANS: A
Response: This option allows you to provide constant supervision of and emotional support for the patient who is suicidal. The precaution also conveys a sense of safety and care by the staff.
Chapter: Suicide

7. Your 15-year-old neighbor, who knows you are a mental health nurse, informs you that he or she has " a friend who is talking about suicide." Your best initial response to the young neighbor is:
A. "Who is it? Another neighbor?"
B. "I have some time. Tell me a little about this friend."
C. "Who else knows? Has this friend told anyone else?"
D. "Your friend needs help right away!"
ANS: B
Response: You display interest in the neighbor's story and allow the young neighbor to share information at his or her own pace. The neighbor is most likely speaking of him or herself and this is an effort to see another's reaction.
Chapter: Suicide

8. You have a 15-year-old neighbor who chooses to speak to you about a friend who is talking about suicide. As you near the end of your conversation with the neighbor, you give the information about the local community mental health center. As a nurse, you know that *all* community mental health facilities must provide:
A. Suicide prevention programs for all age groups
B. Detoxification programs for patients on 72-hour hold
C. Family therapy programs
D. Emergency electroconvulsive therapy (ECT) capability
ANS: A
Response: Suicide prevention for all age groups is a requirement for community mental health agencies. These agencies may also provide detoxification treatment and various therapies; most agencies do not perform ECT.

9. The most important factor for a nurse to assess when evaluating suicide risk in a newly admitted depressed patient is:
A. The patient's plans for the immediate future after discharge
B. How long the person has felt depressed
C. How many personal "problems" the patient lists as stressors
D. How the patient plans to handle the upcoming anniversary of his or her spouse's death
ANS: D
Response: Anniversaries of precipitating events are, often times, when the pain renews itself and when the patient experiences the urge to end his or her own life. Asking the patient about his or her plans for the future is not yet appropriate.
Chapter: Suicide

10. It is the first day of your rotation on the afternoon shift. You hear in a report that one of your patients has "slipped" back into depression. As you make your first rounds, you observe this patient sitting quietly and staring out the window. The patient does not respond when you approach him or her, so you say, therapeutically:
A. "What's the matter? It can't be that bad!"
B. "Pull it together. You are so close to being discharged!"
C. "I understand you are feeling bad. I'd like to help."
D. "What happened? Everything was fine yesterday."
ANS: C
Response: This is a broad opening statement that expresses an implied feeling of the patient's and encourages the patient to verbalize his or her concerns. It also allows the patient to hear your concern for him or her.
Chapter: Suicide

11. A patient confides to you that he or she has been thinking of committing suicide. You realize that this patient
A. Is looking for attention
B. Is looking for help to protect him or herself from acting on the suicidal thoughts
C. Is seeking a shocked reaction from the nurse
D. Considers you, the nurse, to be a "friend"
ANS: B
Response: The patient realizes that there is potential danger in his or her life and is looking for someone to help protect him or her from acting on the thoughts of killing himself or herself.
Chapter: Suicide

12. A "suicide pact" is:
A. A myth of suicide
B. A way to "get even with" parents
C. A written note explaining the reason for the suicide
D. A mutual decision made by members of a peer group to commit suicide
ANS: D
Response: "Suicide pacts" are agreements made by groups of friends or peers who mutually agree to end their lives together.
Chapter: Suicide

13. You have been consistently caring for a patient who is suicidal, but who now tells you, "Nurse, I finally have it all figured out. It's going to be just fine." Your *best* response to this patient is:
A. "I'm so glad to hear that!"
B. "What a relief for you!"
C. "I'm not sure I understand what you mean. Tell me more."
D. "You have an excellent doctor. I knew things would work out in the end!"
ANS: C

Response: This option shows that you are hearing the potential for the patient to actually commit suicide. You ask for clarification from the patient, instead of putting words into the patient's mouth or providing a cliché as a response.
Chapter: Suicide

14. Of the following patient statements, which do nurses recognize as the *highest* risk for a patient to commit suicide?
A. "I've been saving my pain medications for when I really need them. Now that my spouse has left me, and right before the Holidays, I think I really need them."
B. "I told my boss if he fires me, I'll kill myself."
C. "Nobody appreciates the work I do. They'd miss me if I just killed myself and was gone one day."
D. "I really admire people who have enough nerve to kill themselves. I'm not that brave yet."
ANS: A
Response: All of these responses are potentially ones that are said by people contemplating suicide, but option "A" denotes a plan and some definite reasons indicating that this person has planned suicide.
Chapter: Suicide

15. You are caring for a patient who has been treated for major depression, with suicidal tendencies. The patient has progressed in a positive manner, denies feeling suicidal, and is due to be discharged tomorrow. On rounds, you notice that the door to the unit is uncharacteristically open and the patient is not in his or her room. You find the patient hanging by a bed sheet in the chapel. Your reaction to this case is:
A. "Where there is a will, there is a way."
B. The patient was due to be discharged; therefore, he or she was on independent care and allowed to come and go freely.
C. The patient should have been more carefully observed and better anticipated by the nursing staff.
D. The patient no longer showed symptoms of suicidal ideation so there was no need for close supervision.
ANS: C
Response: Nurses know that suicide is more likely to be successful when the patient appears to be energetic and no longer depressed. You should have anticipated this patient's suicidal potential and should not have been falsely lured into the belief that the patient was safe, pending the imminent discharge. Your actions could be interpreted as negligence.
Chapter: Suicide

16. You are working with a 45-year-old male patient who was in middle management. His company has "out-sized" him. A friend of his brings him to your clinic and reports that the patient has been drinking alcohol more frequently than usual. The friend also reports that the patient's father committed suicide and that the patient has been saying, "Dad had the right idea. I think my family would be better off without me, too!" You realize that this patient is at what level of suicide risk?
A. Low
B. Moderate
C. High
D. Very high/imminent
ANS: D
Response: This patient has five of the characteristics of someone who is contemplating suicide. He is at very high risk for suicide at this point.
Chapter: Suicide

17. You are caring for an adolescent patient who has swallowed all of his mother's sleeping and pain pills. The patient has had a gastric lavage and is able to answer questions. The *best* question to ask this patient is:
A. "What are your thoughts right now about hurting yourself?"
B. "Why on earth did you do that?"
C. "Don't you know how much your family loves you and how much they will miss you if you kill yourself?"
D. "This is a very immature way to get attention."
ANS: A
Response: This question is nonjudgmental and allows you to get the patient's perspective on his or her feelings and thoughts. It also helps you assess the suicide risk. This may be one situation where a closed-ended question, such as

"Do you feel like hurting yourself right now?" would be appropriate if the patient is not able to give longer responses.
Chapter: Suicide

18. You are caring for a middle-aged woman who is suffering from major depression and melancholia. She expresses her "failure as a wife and mother" and that she "deserves to die." Your *first* priority to this patient is:
A. Reassure her that she is a very good wife and mother
B. Tell her that her illness is not a punishment and she does not deserve to die
C. Divert her to other activities to get her mind off herself
D. Protect and monitor her for suicidal tendencies
ANS: D
Response: This patient has depressive disorders and feelings of worthlessness. She is at high risk to attempt suicide.
Chapter: Suicide

19. A suicidal patient has been transferred to your unit from the medical floor and asks you why he or she "has to be watched every minute. I have a right to my privacy; I'm an adult and can come and go as I please." The *best* response to this patient is:
A. "Why do you think you are being watched?"
B. "We are concerned that you might attempt to seriously hurt yourself."
C. "It shouldn't bother you if you have nothing to hide from us."
D. "This is a direct order from your doctor."
ANS: B
Response: The physician may well have ordered the transfer and direct observation, but that would not make a difference to the patient. The *best* response for a nurse in this situation is to honestly tell the patient about the staff's concerns for the patient's safety and well-being.
Chapter: Suicide

20. A 65-year-old female patient is admitted to your unit following an unsuccessful suicide attempt. She has a long history of depressive disorders. Medication and therapy have been unsuccessful for her. She is scheduled to begin ECT. You patient teaching for this patient should include:
A. "ECT will finally cure your symptoms!"
B. "You can expect some permanent memory loss from the ECT."
C. "Only one of these treatments if usually required to eliminate depressive symptoms."
D. "You will most likely feel confused for a few hours when you wake up from the ECT."
ANS: D
Response: Confusion, although usually temporary, is a major side effect of the ECT. You will need to keep the patient oriented following this procedure.
Chapter: Suicide

21. Which of the groups listed below is the lowest risk group, according to current data, to commit suicide?
A. Married, white females
B. Minority groups
C. Elderly people (especially white men)
D. Adolescents
ANS: A
Response: Married, white females are currently the lowest group of those listed. Researchers are not positive, but the current thought is that this group may attempt suicide, but either cannot or will not carry out the act.
Chapter: Suicide

Aging Population

1. Which of the following statements is *most* accurate regarding aging?
A. Everyone ages at the same rate.
B. Aging is a very individual process.
C. Aging begins at age 65.
D. Everyone over age 60 is considered old.

ANS: B
Response: Aging is different for all individuals and begins at different ages for all individuals. There are many myths associated with the aging process.
Chapter: Aging Population

2. Nurses know that the occurrence of chronic illness is highest in:
A. School-aged children
B. Adolescents
C. Middle adulthood
D. Older adulthood
ANS: D
Response: Older adults have the highest incidence of chronic illness.
Chapter: Aging Population

3. Because of some of the changes associated with the aging process, nurses understand that elderly people have a high incidence of hip fractures because elderly people are:
A. Forgetful and careless
B. Inactive
C. Subject to bone decalcification
D. Stubborn
ANS: C
Response: Decalcification of bones, as part of the aging process in elderly people (especially in elderly women), is a major cause of hip and pathological spinal fractures.
Chapter: Aging Population

4. Mr. Burns, who is 80-years-old, is scheduled for cataract surgery. You are responsible for his preoperative and postoperative teaching and he expresses his fear and anxiety to you. He says, "I'm just too old for this. You can't teach an old dog new tricks." You respond to his concerns by saying:
A. "You seem concerned about your surgery, Mr. Burns. I'm here to help if you'd like to talk about it."
B. "You're only as old as you feel, Mr. Burns!"
C. "You might surprise yourself, Mr. Burns!"
D. "You have to learn this or your doctor can't do the surgery and your vision will not improve, Mr. Burns."
ANS: A
Response: Your response tells the patient that you hear his concerns and that you have the time and the desire to discuss these concerns with him.
Chapter: Aging Population

5. Mrs. Black, a 65-year-old widow, is admitted to the medical floor with an exacerbation of her congestive heart failure (CHF). She has been on this unit before, but the CHF is worse now than it was on previous admissions. You know that besides her physical situation, Mrs. Black is also at risk for:
A. Depression
B. Schizophrenia
C. Delusions
D. Borderline personality disorder
ANS: A
Response: Her advancing age, her status of being a widow, and advancement of her CHF are strong indicators that she is also a candidate for depression.
Chapter: Aging Population

6. An elderly patient who is having an annual physical examination at the clinic states, "Speak up! Everyone just mumbles these days. Can't you speak up?" You understand that this patient is:
A. Cranky
B. Deaf
C. Mentally ill
D. Experiencing hearing loss associated with aging

ANS: D
Response: This patient seems to have diminished hearing. This partial hearing loss is a part of aging, and may be either natural or pathological.
Chapter: Aging Population

7. When planning care for an elderly patient, a safety consideration the nurse must address is:
A. Clothing must be long and loose
B. Keep the patient in a specific, confined area at all times
C. Provide adequate lighting
D. Turn the water temperature up, because the patient is always cold
ANS: C
Response: Visual acuity decreases with age. Providing adequate lighting is mandatory for promoting the safety of elderly patients.
Chapter: Aging Population

8. An 80-year-old patient is brought to the urgent care center. The patient is unconscious and the physician suspects a cerebrovascular accident (CVA/stroke). You are assisting, so your first priority for this patient is to:
A. Perform the Glasgow Coma Scale
B. Perform CPR
C. Call the family
D. Maintain patency of airway
ANS: D
Response: In this case, your first priority is physical, not emotional, safety. Patency of airway is the priority for this patient.
Chapter: Aging Population

9. Mr. Gone is a 79-year-old patient who is being discharged from your hospital. He lives independently, but has periods of forgetfulness. It is important to include his family when teaching about his medications primarily to:
A. Provide a reference and support system for him
B. Convince his family that they should go to his house daily to give his medications
C. Encourage him to move to a nursing home or an assisted living facility
D. Gain the family's approval for the medications
ANS: A
Response: The support of the family is required, but not their approval. It is important that they do not undermine treatment. Education does not ensure approval, but it usually improves support.
Chapter: Aging Population

10.Nurses expect that an elderly patient who is experiencing presbycusis, (hearing loss associated with aging), would:
A. Have copious amounts of cerumen in the ear
B. Have more trouble hearing female voices than male voices
C. Have fluid behind the eardrum
D. Have ear surgery
ANS: B
Response: High-pitched sounds are typically more difficult to hear than low-pitched sounds in presbycusis; therefore, it may be beneficial to have male caregivers administer to patients with presbycusis when possible.
Chapter: Aging Population

11. All of the following are myths about aging *except*:
A. Old people are senile.
B. Old people are not alone or isolated.
C. Old people are all crabby.
D. Old people dislike young people.
ANS: B

Response: The "myth" or "false statement" is that all elderly people *are* alone and isolated. Some elderly people are, but many are social and living and participating in their communities.
Chapter: Aging Population

12. A basic attitude about aging in western culture is:
A. Elderly people have little to contribute to society.
B. Elderly people are held in high honor.
C. Elderly people are good resource people.
D. Elderly people have valuable skills.
ANS: A
Response: Western culture has the attitude that older adults have made their contribution to society and have little else to offer.
Chapter: Aging Population

13. You are caring for a 70-year-old patient who had a stroke and are concerned with the emotional and physical well-being of that patient. The emotional responses of a patient who has suffered a left CVA would be affected by:
A. The patient's ability to understand the condition
B. The location of the lesion
C. The patient's personality type before the stroke
D. The relationship of the patient and his or her spouse
ANS: C
Response: All of these may be factors, but the main influence on a patient's emotional recovery after a stroke is the type of personality and coping skills the patient had prior to the stroke.
Chapter: Aging Population

14. Caring for the elderly patient can be challenging. Nurses must be aware of their feelings about the aging process in order to:
A. Joke with the patients
B. Be more sympathetic
C. Project the "right" attitude toward others
D. Be more therapeutic
ANS: D
Response: Option "D" implies that nurses who care for the elderly population are aware that this population has special needs and that special techniques in physical and emotional care may be required of nurses.
Chapter: Aging Population

15. When providing care for elderly people who are in nursing homes, nurses understand that a major consideration for the elderly patient is:
A. Promoting personal hygiene and self-esteem
B. Making important decisions for the elderly patient
C. Insisting on doing all tasks for the elderly patient
D. Allowing the elderly patient to do what he or she wishes
ANS: A
Response: Promoting hygiene and self-esteem are two of many important considerations that nurses must make when planning care for elderly patients
Chapter: Aging Population

16. When caring for elderly patients who have had a stroke, nurses will assist the patient toward independence by:
A. Establishing many long-term goals with the patient
B. Praising the patient's small successes
C. Immediately correcting errors in the patient's task completion
D. Showing the patient other patients who worked hard and "got better"
ANS: B
Response: Small successes are very huge for the patient who has had a stroke. Recognition and praise of the patient's success reinforces the patient's work and encourages further interest in improving his or her capacity.

17. You are admitting an elderly patient who is undergoing testing to rule out or diagnose Alzheimer's dementia. During your interview, the patient informs you that "You ask too many questions. Leave me alone. I don't want to be here anyway." The *best* therapeutic nursing response to this patient is:
A. "Oh, come on, now. You don't really feel that way."
B. "That's the way hospitals are. We just ask questions all of the time!"
C. "Your daughter will be upset with you if you don't answer these questions."
D. "You sound upset. Would you like to rest a while? I'll come back in an hour."
ANS: D
Response: This response shows your concern for the patient's emotional well-being and conveys the knowledge that you understand that, often times, elderly people have a decreased tolerance to stimulation and need a break.
Chapter: Aging Population

18. A 70-year-old male patient comes to the clinic stating that the allergy medication he bought at the drug store makes him "goofy." He says he takes the medication "according to the directions, but I feel sleepy and confused when I take it." He is otherwise alert and oriented and lives in his own home with his wife, cat, and dog. The nurse obtaining this information considers that:
A. Elderly people often require a lower than usual dose of medication
B. Elderly people usually cannot understand the dosing directions on over-the-counter medications
C. Elderly people usually require a higher than usual dose of medication
D. He has probably taken the medication with another one that is contraindicated
ANS: A
Response: Elderly people have slower metabolisms. They often eat less than younger adults and get less exercise. They require less than usual dosages of medication in many cases.
Chapter: Aging Population

19. Charles is an 80-year-old man newly added to your home-care assignment. He is diagnosed with CHF and type 2 diabetes mellitus. He has decubitus ulcers on his buttocks and heels. He is also being treated for mild depression, for which the doctor has him on a full dose of fluoxetine (Prozac). You are concerned about the dose of Prozac because you know:
A. Elderly people should not take antidepressant medications
B. Elderly people commonly need as little as 25 percent of the usual adult dose of a medication
C. Elderly people are in a risk group for suicide and should take a higher than usual adult dose of Prozac
D. The side effects of Prozac may allow Charles to forget to take his insulin
ANS: B
Response: It is not uncommon for older adults to require as little as 25 percent of the recommended adult dose of many medications.
Chapter: Aging Population

20. The best nursing intervention for you as the licensed practical nurse/licensed vocational nurse caring for Charles is:
A. Do nothing and see how the Prozac works for him
B. Tell Charles to stop taking the medication
C. Call the doctor and state your concern
D. None of the above
ANS: C
Response: Because nurses are ultimately responsible for administering medications safely, it would be appropriate for the nurse to call the doctor to discuss the dose.
Chapter: Aging Population

Victims of Abuse

1. When teaching about child abuse, nurses explain that *assault* is defined as:

A. Actual harm or threats of harm to another person
B. A legal term for wrongful harm to another person's property
C. A legal term for rape
D. Physical force against another person without justification
ANS: A
Response: "Assault" is actual or implied bodily harm to another person.
Chapter: Victims of Abuse

2. Laws pertaining to abuse of children or any vulnerable person dictate that:
A. Anyone who suspects abuse is bound to report it
B. Physicians must report actual or suspected abuse
C. Nurses must report actual or suspected abuse
D. Nurses/physicians only report actual abuse
ANS: A
Response: All people, not only health care providers, are legally responsible for reporting actual or suspected abuse of any vulnerable person regardless of their age.
Chapter: Victims of Abuse

3. Nurses would expect that a nonthreatening form of therapy for a child who has been sexually abused would be:
A. Systematic desensitization
B. Group therapy
C. Art or play therapy
D. Rational emotive therapy
ANS: C
Response: Offering a child art or play therapy gives the child a nonthreatening way of expressing the thoughts and feelings surrounding the abuse, as well as assisting in ways to help begin their problem solving.
Chapter: Victims of Abuse

4. The main goal of a nurse when caring for a child or adolescent who is in crisis is:
A. Let the patient "work it out," because adults "don't understand anyway"
B. Explore the underlying cause of the crisis with the patient
C. Stop the abusive situation
D. Immediately report the situation as child abuse
ANS: B
Response: This crisis situation stops short of stating that the child or adolescent is, in fact, being abused. Option "B" allows the nurse to explore the causes in an open-ended manner.
Chapter: Victims of Abuse

5. A patient states she is having flashbacks about a rape that happened several months ago. She becomes dyspneic and diaphoretic. Her heart rate increases to 120 beats per minute. You decide that an appropriate focus for the patient's nursing diagnosis is:
A. Ineffective individual coping
B. Knowledge deficit
C. Impaired circulatory function: actual
D. Panic
ANS: D
Response: The patient exhibits symptoms of panic resulting from the stress of the rape.
Chapter: Victims of Abuse

6. You are caring for a 2-year-old who screams and cries uncontrollably after parental visits. The child's crying wakes the other children, so you choose to move the child in his or her crib to the supply closet for a half-hour. Legally:
A. You are correct, because children need to learn appropriate behavior limits.
B. You are correct, because the rights of the other children were being infringed upon.

189

C. You are incorrect, because there was no threat of direct danger to this child or the other children in the ward.
D. You are incorrect, because the time limit you chose was a little too long to keep the child separated from the others.
ANS: C
Response: It is legally unacceptable to segregate patients if there is no threat of danger either to that patient or to the others in the vicinity.
Chapter: Victims of Abuse

7. A 4-year-old who has chickenpox will not stop scratching despite your numerous attempts to stop him or her "or else I'll have to tie your hands down!" By responding this way to a patient, you
A. Exhibit behaviors that are within the definition of "assault"
B. Try to talk to the child at his or her own level of understanding
C. Display responsibility in performing your tasks
D. Choose to protect the child's skin and explain this to him or her in a professional manner
ANS: A
Response: Your response sounds threatening and would most likely be legally interpreted as "assault."
Chapter: Victims of Abuse

8. Martina, who is pregnant, arrives at your urgent care center after her husband has battered her. Women who are physically abused most frequently present first at:
A. Obstetrics clinics
B. Emergency rooms
C. Women's shelters
D. Mental health clinics
ANS: A
Response: Most women who are abused will not bring themselves to a clinic unless they are concerned for their unborn child. For this reason, it is most common to see women who are battered presenting first at their obstetrics clinic.
Chapter: Victims of Abuse

9. A battered woman in the shelter states that she "is afraid to go home because he drinks. That's when he gets violent and he beats me." You are able to provide the following information to this patient:
A. "If you can get him to quit drinking, the beating will stop."
B. "Alcohol use can increase the chances of abuse."
C. "People who use alcohol almost always end up as abusers."
D. "He's just using the alcohol as an excuse to beat you."
ANS: B
Response: Alcohol use and abuse greatly increase the chances of violence against another because it lowers inhibitions and alters thought processes.
Chapter: Victims of Abuse

10. Which of the following adult behaviors would indicate the occurrence of nonsexual physical abuse received as a child?
A. Slowed cognitive development
B. Poor communication skills
C. Discomfort upon hearing children cry
D. Echopraxia
ANS: C
Response: Older children and adults who were abused as children often become obviously uncomfortable when they hear other children crying.
Chapter: Victims of Abuse

11. Women of low-socioeconomic groups have more frequently been identified as being battered, than women of middle- or high-socioeconomic groups. Which of the following choices offers the best rationale for this statement?

A. Men from low-socioeconomic groups are more violent.
B. Men from middle- and high-socioeconomic groups are less violent.
C. Women from low-socioeconomic groups more frequently put themselves into dangerous situations.
D. Women from middle- and high-socioeconomic groups conceal their battering.
ANS: D
Response: Women from middle- to high-socioeconomic groups usually have more private medical care and the means available to prevent them from reporting their battering.
Chapter: Victims of Abuse

12. You are working nights in the free clinic. A woman is brought in by a female friend. According to the friend, the woman has been raped. The *first* nursing intervention for this patient is:
A. Reassure her that she is safe
B. Get the rape kit and perform the examination
C. Ask her who did this to her
D. Call an attorney for her
ANS: A
Response: It is vital that a woman (or man) who has been raped feels safe in your institution. Performing the examination is crucial, but patients will be more willing to cooperate with the examination if they feel safe.
Chapter: Victims of Abuse

13. A person who has just been raped is in crisis. "Crisis intervention" is a short-term treatment. Nurses understand that crisis will usually be resolved in:
A. 1 to 2 days
B. 1 to 2 weeks
C. 4 to 6 weeks
D. 1 year
ANS: C
Response: Crisis is generally resolved within 4 to 6 weeks. Depending on the cause of the crisis, therapy may be required to deal with the underlying issues, but the actual stage of the crisis will have been handled.
Chapter: Victims of Abuse

14. Nurses must care for the abused person, as well as the abuser. You are caring for a middle-aged man who is under medical and psychiatric care for molesting a 7-year-old girl. You inform him that dinner is being served in the dining room. He tells you to leave and that he does not want anyone to see him or "know what I did." You respond:
A. "You will need to face people sooner or later."
B. "You are here for treatment of an illness, not judgment of an action."
C. "I guess I wouldn't want to been seen either. You may stay here."
D. "Only the staff knows the reason for your admission."
ANS: B
Response: Option "B" conveys your understanding of the patient's feelings. Your response neither supports nor reprimands the behavior. You only state the fact that this is a person in need of medical and psychiatric care and that the staff is there to provide that care.
Chapter: Victims of Abuse

15. You are caring for a 6-year-old boy who has been allegedly abused by his mother. During his mother's visits, you expect her to have which of the following characteristics?
A. A strong and loving relationship with her parents
B. Middle-class socioeconomic level
C. A history of being abused as a child
D. Realistic expectations of herself and her child
ANS: C
Response: There is a strong correlation between being an abuser and having been abused.
Chapter: Victims of Abuse

16. You are a nurse who is also volunteering with your community's women's abuse program. A woman tells you that she is afraid her 3-year-old saw the assault. You must be aware that:
A. Some states consider that child to also be abused
B. A 3-year-old will probably not remember the assault, so the woman does not need to worry
C. There must be physical contact with the child in order for the abuser's actions to be considered "abuse."
D. All of the above
ANS: A
Response: Some states have either passed legislation or are discussing legislation that considers children who witness abuse, either visual or auditory, also to be abused. You would need to report your findings to the child protection agency in your state. It is important for nurses to be keenly aware of the laws in their state that pertain to children who witness abuse.
Chapter: Victims of Abuse

17. Besides the home, the area that seems to be growing most rapidly in frequency for reports of violence is:
A. Shopping malls
B. Sporting events
C. On the road (road rage)
D. Workplace
ANS: D
Response: Workplace violence is the fastest-growing area of abuse. Road rage is also growing in frequency, but because workplace violence includes a broad range of circumstances (e.g., verbal abuse, hostile workplace, supervisor issues), the workplace is running second to the home for frequency of reports of violence.
Chapter: Victims of Abuse